Sexuality, Sexual and Gender Identities and Intimacy Research in Social Work and Social Care

Until now, sexuality has been treated as a specialist topic or area of specialist social work practice. This book cuts across all areas of the discipline. It examines the relationship between sexuality, sexual identities and intimacies and the life course, and showcases a range of issues pertinent to social work through these lenses. It opens up new possibilities for better understanding sexuality in social work, and contains empirical work and theorising about sexuality, intimacy and gender not currently found in a traditional course on life course theory and practice.

The chapters position new areas of scholarship in sexuality including trans perspectives, masculinities, bisexuality and the voices of other gender and sexual minority populations within a life course trajectory. Empirical research picks up on the broader public health and well-being agenda with a strong focus on challenging normative theories to promote human rights and justice for marginalised individuals and groups.

Sexuality, Sexual and Gender Identities and Intimacy Research in Social Work and Social Care will significantly enhance any core texts on life course theory and practice, anti-oppression and anti-discriminatory theories for professionals. It should be considered essential reading for academics, practitioners and undergraduate and postgraduate students.

Priscilla Dunk-West is Senior Lecturer in social work at Flinders University, Australia. Her practice background was in London where she worked in child protection with families, children and young people before specialising in sexual health in Australia. Her research focuses on social work and sexuality, everyday sexuality and intimacy, long-term relationships and positive post separation parenting.

Trish Hafford-Letchfield is a qualified nurse, social worker and educator who has been working in higher education since 2003. Trish is Professor of Social Care at Middlesex University and Social Work Research Fellow at the University of Stellenbosch, in South Africa. Her research interests are diverse including sexualities and sexual identities, older people from marginalised communities, equality issues in health and social care and the use of the arts in education and practice to promote community engagement.

Sexuality, Sexual and Gender Identities and Intimacy Research in Social Work and Social Care

A Lifecourse Epistemology

Edited by Priscilla Dunk-West and Trish Hafford-Letchfield

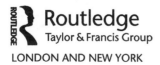

Routledge
Taylor & Francis Group

LONDON AND NEW YORK

First published 2018 by Routledge

2 Park Square, Milton Park, Abingdon, Oxfordshire OX14 4RN
52 Vanderbilt Avenue, New York, NY 10017

Routledge is an imprint of the Taylor & Francis Group, an informa business

First issued in paperback 2020

British Library Cataloguing-in-Publication Data
A catalogue record for this book is available from the British Library

Library of Congress Cataloging-in-Publication Data
Names: Dunk-West, Priscilla, editor. | Hafford-Letchfield, Trish, editor.
Title: Sexuality, sexual and gender identities and intimacy research in social work and social care: a lifecourse epistemology / edited by Priscilla Dunk-West and Trish Hafford-Letchfield.
Description: 1st Edition. | New York: Routledge, 2018. | Includes bibliographical references and index.
Identifiers: LCCN 2017053994
Subjects: LCSH: Social service—Research. |
Social service—Practice. | Sexism. | Sex. | Gender identity.
Classification: LCC HV11 .S4759 2018 | DDC 362.89/6—dc23
LC record available at https://lccn.loc.gov/2017053994

ISBN: 978-1-138-22587-9 (hbk)
ISBN: 978-0-367-59179-3 (pbk)

Typeset in Times New Roman
by codeMantra

Contents

List of figures and tables   vii
Foreword   ix
Acknowledgements   xiii
List of contributors   xv

1 **Sexuality, sexual and gender identities and intimacy research in social work and social care: what does the life course lens have to offer?**   1
TRISH HAFFORD-LETCHFIELD AND PRISCILLA DUNK-WEST

2 **Gender non-conforming children, trans youth and their family: identifying best evidences and practices for social work interventions**   11
ANNIE PULLEN SANSFAÇON

3 **Combatting homophobic and transphobic bullying in schools through family engagement**   27
TRISH HAFFORD-LETCHFIELD, CHRISTINE COCKER,
PETER RYAN, MARY MARTIN, ROSALIND SCOTT
AND SARAH CARR

4 **Intimacy in young women's friendships: symbols and rituals**   49
KATIE LETCHFIELD AND TRISH HAFFORD-LETCHFIELD

5 **Home and 'hood': middle-aged gay men's stories of homes and neighbourhoods**   69
PAUL SIMPSON

6 **Transgender people negotiating intimate relationships**   86
DAMIEN W. RIGGS, HENRY VON DOUSSA AND JENNIFER POWER

7 'Out' and about at work: institutionalised heteronormativity on
relationships and employment 101
ALFONSO PEZZELLA

8 Measuring relationship quality in an international study:
exploratory and confirmatory factor validity 121
JILL M. CHONODY, JACQUI GABB, MIKE KILLIAN AND
PRISCILLA DUNK-WEST

9 Bisexuality and ageing: why it matters for social work practice 142
KATHRYN ALMACK, REBECCA L. JONES AND
RACHAEL M. SCICLUNA

10 Single women living alone in later life: evidence from
Understanding Society data 155
HAFIZ T.A. KHAN, TRISH HAFFORD-LETCHFIELD AND
NICKY LAMBERT

11 Stories of intimacy and sexuality in later life: Solo women speak 176
NICKY LAMBERT, TRISH HAFFORD-LETCHFIELD,
HAFIZ T.A. KHAN, DOMINIQUE BRADY, ELLOUISE LONG
AND LISA CLARKE

12 Sexuality, gender and intimacy, reflecting on professional practice 197
PRISCILLA DUNK-WEST AND TRISH HAFFORD-LETCHFIELD

Index 203

List of figures and tables

Figures

3.1   Snapshot of work generated by the teams   40
8.1   Confirmatory factor analysis: item loadings (n = 4,066).
       Items correspond to item list in Table 8.5   136
10.1 Path diagram showing linkages between selected variables
       considered in the study about here   160
11.1 Thematic analysis of the survey qualitative data   183

Tables

3.1   Examples of good practice from the school participants data   35
3.2   Structure of the workshop programme   39
4.1   Characteristics of sample   53
4.2   Characteristics of rituals and symbols from the data   54
5.1   Recruitment of participants   73
5.2   Participants' social class   74
8.1   Socio-demographic description of sample   132
8.2   Ethnicity by country   133
8.3   Exploratory factor analysis: factor loadings (n = 4,066)   134
8.4   Confirmatory factor analysis: model fit indices (n = 4,066)   136
8.5   Final relationship quality (RQ) scale   136
10.1 Characteristics of general population as well as study
       population about here   160
10.2 Cross-tabulations between characteristics of older women
       in the household about here   165
10.3 Logistic regression result displays the important factors
       influencing the dependent variables   167
11.1 Survey questions   180

List of figures and tables

Figures

Tables

Foreword

When I was a young adolescent struggling to make sense of my sexuality and identity in the late 1970s—long before the age of online resources at our fingertips, long before the possibility of marriage equality and long before I would even be legal in most countries—I did what many queer people did in that generation: I went to the library. I went there in order to read up on myself, to make sense of my very confused experiences and to try to find a language to explain who I was. Because of the terrible shame associated with being caught in a public place reading those few resources, I began to purchase these books so I could read them at home. I even remember naively thinking that I could create my own library of queer resources, keep up with all the newly published books and ideas and create my own private world where I was normal.

Things have changed. Clandestine trips to the library have been replaced by devices we carry around in our pockets and purses that find queer resources in an instant. I can't imagine a private collection that could keep up with all the books on sexuality, gender, identity, HIV and queer theory that have exploded in the last generation. Transmen and transwomen are in the daily news. Hollywood (and Bollywood and Nollywood) actors and singers, athletes and artists, prime ministers and politicians around the world publicly identify themselves as sexual or gender minorities. At this writing, all or parts of 24 countries have marriage equality, and more are on the way. Still, though (at this writing), I am illegal in 76 countries, many of them members of the former British Empire. In many places of the world, queer people are still being stigmatised, arrested, tortured and killed, simply for daring to be who they are (and even who they are alleged to be). Gender non-conforming people are subject to what is ironically called 'corrective' rape, under the theory that once lesbians and gender non-binary people have had a taste of heteromale violence they will want more of it. There is certainly much, much more work to be done. But oh, how far we have come to make much of the world a safer, healthier and gayer place for sexual and gender minorities.

We are still trying to make sense of our sexualities, identities and intimate relationships. The volume you hold in your hand (or are reading on a screen!) continues the necessary work of exploring and theorising about all the ways we come to terms with ourselves throughout our entire lives. Becoming aware of the enduring impact of bullying, exclusion, oppression and violence, either by state or private actors, is a lifelong task for most of us. What cisgender heteronormative oppression has done, however, is brought all kinds and colours and flavours of sexual and gender minorities together not only to support each other, but to challenge privileged notions of normalcy that are used against us. We recognise now that we are affected by this bullying and oppression throughout our entire lives, and we emancipate ourselves by naming and rejecting these notions that still shape so much of our lived experience. There is a group of queer theorists who claim we are living in a post-gay world, where identity labels are no longer meaningful. Perhaps that is true: but we are still living in a world where sexual and gender minorities must differentiate ourselves from the dominant cisgender hetero-discourse. Once we are able do that, we begin to see and understand the world and ourselves differently. We begin the process of rejecting the inherited epistemology of oppression, and form our own radically subjective epistemologies which validate truths and norms through our own lived experiences as queer persons. We engage in this process throughout our entire lives—from the moment we become aware of our difference until the moment of our final breath. For some of us that process begins when we are quite young. For others, who may not have had a way to articulate their experience of difference until later in their lives, this process may begin later. Until the end of heteronormative cisgender patriarchy, however, we will always be aware of ourselves as different: the ways we live in the world and validate truth will be different: at home, in school, at work or in older age; in family groups, in relationships and in our individual experiences. This book invites us to interrogate notions of self, relationship and family, and to develop new understandings of those familiar terms.

It is the task of the social worker to understand and to work with persons in the contexts of their environments. People and environments are constantly changing, so the work of social workers is always dynamic, both in the sense of always changing, and of being powerful. Social justice is at the core of what we do. If environments are oppressive or dangerous, social workers around the world must work to make those environments less oppressive and less dangerous. We do this through all the usual tools available to us as social workers, in all the practice settings in which social workers do their work. We do this in the same ways that we challenge gender inequality, racism, colonialism and all the multifarious forces that collude to marginalise and vulnerabilise people. As a social work educator, I hope that my colleagues and their students will take advantage of this book and ensure that the topics that it addresses are in their course curricula. I hope that social workers in practice will make it a part of their continuing professional development plans. The material covered in this book belongs in every social work curriculum so that students, beginning practitioners and experienced social workers are prepared to practice competently with all persons. No single book can do everything, but this book is another way for us to learn and to equip ourselves to work for social justice in the world.

It is a privilege for me to be associated in some small way with this important project. Over the course of my life I have become increasingly radicalised as I have come to make sense of my sexuality and identity. I learned that it was not my sexuality that was confused or required explaining: it was the world around me that told me that I was mad, bad, sad, sinful, selfish and sick, and I learned to challenge those labels. I learned that none of those stigmatising stereotypes are true, and it is important to remind ourselves of that again and again. The editors and contributing authors have provided us with an important opportunity to learn more from the lived experiences of sexual and gender minorities, so that social workers and other helping professionals can learn to make those life experiences both more powerful and more meaningful.

Dr Mark Henrickson
Professor of Social Work,
Auckland, Aotearoa New Zealand

Acknowledgements

We wish to thank all the inspiring colleagues, many of whom have become good friends from the *International Sexuality in Social Work Network*. May the activism continue, and if you don't already belong, please join this excellent network via JISCMAIL or Facebook. A special thanks from Trish to dear friends Christine Cocker and Kate Leonard and to my lovely family, Ted, Katie, Mum, Anne, Guy, Nathan, Claudia, Imogen and Theodore. Thanks to our new-found USA Johnston kin who make life very special. Heartfelt thanks from Priscilla to her support crew—Penny, Kylie and of course to Blake and Paxton: the dudes.

We wish to thank Sage Publications for permission to reproduce the following material in Chapter 8 of this book: Jill M. Chonody, Jacqui Gabb, Mike Killian, Priscilla Dunk-West (2016) 'Measuring Relationship Quality in an International Study: Exploratory and Confirmatory Factor Validity', *Journal of Research on Social Work Practice*. Article first published online: August 3, 2016. https://doi.org/10.1177/1049731516631120.

List of contributors

Kathryn Almack is Professor of Health, Young People and Family Lives at the University of Hertfordshire. She has undertaken a number of research projects exploring and addressing the care needs and experiences of older LGBT people in later and towards the end of life. This includes a two-year study funded by the Marie Curie Research Programme, The Last Outing (2013–2015) and subsequent studies also funded by Marie Curie. Findings from this body of work have been used to develop new resources for policy makers and health and social care professionals. Kathryn was also co-applicant for an ESRC funded seminar series—Older LGBT People: Minding the Knowledge Gaps. She has been involved in a number of consultations and action research projects with lesbian, gay, bisexual and transgender (LGBT) people and those who work with them, in collaboration with key end of life care organisations in the UK.

Dominique Brady is a registered social worker and works in London. She has a special interest in working with older people and has worked in hospital discharge and admission avoidance teams. Dominique has participated in research studies to promote the evidence base for working in adult social care and contributes to social work education.

Sarah Carr is Associate Professor of Mental Health and has nearly 20 years' experience of research, knowledge management and policy analysis in mental health and social care. Sarah has particular expertise in service user participation, co-production and equality and has published widely on these topics. She was a member of the NIHR INVOLVE standing committee, supporting public and patient involvement in research. She has lived experience of mental health service use. She specialises in personalisation (person-centred practice and personal budgets), the social aspects of mental health, user and specialist community organisations, evidence-based practice, policy and research analysis and literature reviewing. Sarah holds Honorary academic posts including Senior Lecturer at the School for Social Policy, Birmingham and Visiting Fellow at the School of Social Policy and Social Work at York where she co-chairs the Lived Experience Advisory Panel at the International Centre for Mental Health Social Research.

Jill M. Chonody is an Associate Professor of Social Work at Boise State University and an Adjunct Research Fellow at the University of South Australia. She holds a PhD in social work and is a licensed clinical social worker. Her primary research interests include the study of attitudes toward older adults among social work students, faculty and practitioners and how curriculum can address biases that promote social injustice against older people, those that identify as LGBTQ and women. She is also interested in the way that creativity can be used in research, in particular photographic techniques, and scale development to measure negative attitudes toward those who may be vulnerable or oppressed. Dr Chonody has presented her research both nationally and internationally and has over 40 published articles and book chapters.

Lisa Clarke, PhD teaches research design and methods to undergraduate and postgraduate students in the Department of Law and Politics at Middlesex University. Prior to teaching, Lisa worked as a research fellow on a range of community and student centred projects. Her research interests focus on using technology to enhance learning, and her recent research projects include digital storytelling as an effective teaching, learning and assessment tool and conducting collaborative research with students to evaluate experiences of using computer-assisted qualitative data analysis software (CAQDAS) in teaching and learning. Lisa also runs computer-based CPD courses in qualitative data analysis in the UK, Eastern and Central Europe and the Middle East.

Christine Cocker is a qualified social worker and a Senior Lecturer in Social Work at the University of East Anglia, Norwich, UK. She is an independent member of a local authority adoption panel. Christine completed her social work training in New Zealand in the 1980s. She had worked as a social worker and a social work manager in an inner London local authority and at a national voluntary sector consultation service prior to moving into academia. Her research and publications are predominantly in the area of social work with looked after children, child protection and lesbian and gay fostering and adoption. Amongst her many publications are: Social Work with Lesbians and Gay Men (2011) with Helen Cosis Brown, published by Sage, and an edited book with Trish Hafford Letchfield (2014) Rethinking Anti-Discriminatory and Anti-Oppressive Theories for Social Work Practice, with Palgrave.

Henry von Doussa lives in Melbourne and works as a social researcher for La Trobe and Monash Universities. Much of his work is in the areas of sexuality and sexual health. He recently worked on the longitudinal research project 'Work, Love, Play: Understanding resilience in same-sex parented families' undertaken by The Bouverie Centre in Melbourne. Henry currently works on a randomised control trial of a family focused intervention for families where a parent has a mental illness.

Priscilla Dunk-West is Senior Lecturer in social work at Flinders University, Australia. Her practice background was in London where she worked in child protection with families, children and young people before specialising in sexual health in Australia. Her research focuses on social work and sexuality, everyday sexuality and intimacy, long-term relationships and positive post separation parenting. She is the author of How to be a Social Worker: A Critical Guide for Students (Palgrave Macmillan), co-author with Fiona Verity of Sociological Social Work (Ashgate) and co-author with Fiona Verity of the forthcoming book Practising Social Work Sociologically: A Theoretical Approach for New Times (Palgrave Macmillan).

Jacqui Gabb is Professor of Sociology at the Open University. Her critically acclaimed methodological expertise and interdisciplinary research in the fields of family and sexuality studies have established her as a leading national and international figure, research excellence that is evidenced by world-class research outputs, track record in prestigious RCUK (Research Councils, UK) funding including the Economic and Social Research Council and British Academy, high profile impact and public engagement activities and measures of external esteem. Professor Gabb is the recipient of the BSA Philip Abrams Memorial Prize, 2009, the Evelyn Gillian Research Impact Award (2016) and winner of the BSA Philip Abrams Memorial Prize (2009) for best sole-authored first book in Sociology, for her book Researching Intimacy in Families.

Trish Hafford-Letchfield is Professor of Social Care at Middlesex University London, UK and is a qualified nurse, social worker, educator and manager. Trish's research interests are in equality and diversity issues and particularly in promoting the engagement of older people from marginalised communities in social care. She has especially promoted co-production in her research including arts-based methods and much of her research aims to have a direct impact on professional practice.

Rebecca L. Jones is a Senior Lecturer in Health in the School of Health, Wellbeing and Social Care at The Open University, UK. Her research interests centre on ageing, sexuality and sexuality in later life, especially bisexuality and ageing. Previous research projects have focused on age discrimination, the housing needs of older people with visual impairments, how people imagine their own ageing and later life, normative and non-normative life courses, the ageing of LGBT (lesbians, gay men, bisexual people and transgender) people and LGBT issues in health and social care. She is a founding member of BiUK (www.biuk.org) and co-author of The Bisexuality Report.

Hafiz T.A. Khan is Professor of Public Health at University of West London, UK and an associated research fellow at the Oxford Institute of Population Ageing, University of Oxford in the UK. He trained as a health statistician and has worked in public health and demography over the last

25 years. Hafiz has worked with several reputable institutions internationally including Scotland, Austria, Singapore, Bangladesh and India. He teaches applied statistics, quantitative methods, public Health, demography and health economics. His research interests include the demography of ageing, health and well-being in later life with special focus on loneliness, multi-morbidity, long-term care and support provisions with over 100 research articles in journals, working papers and book chapters on health and population related issues. He has co-authored two books "Research Methods for Business and Social Science", Sage, 2007 and 2014. He is volunteering as trustee at Age UK Oxfordshire, UK.

Mike Killian is an Assistant Professor of Social Work at the School of Social Work at the University of Texas at Arlington (USA) Research Faculty at Children's Medical Center of Dallas (USA) and a Research Affiliate of the Tilda Goldberg Centre for Social Work and Social Care at the University of Bedfordshire (UK). His interests include social work practice with children and families in the area of paediatric health and child welfare/protection as well as advanced statistical and quantitative methodology in social work research.

Nicky Lambert is an Associate Professor (Practice) at Middlesex University, where she is Director of Teaching and Learning for Mental Health, Social Work and Integrative Medicine. She is registered as a Specialist Practitioner (NMC) and is a Senior Teaching Fellow (SFHEA). Nicky has worked across a range of mental health services both in the UK and internationally, supporting staff and practice development in acute and mental health trusts, councils, businesses and charities. She is on the editorial board for Mental Health Nursing and is a Trustee for West Hampstead Women's centre. Nicky has a professional Twitter feed: https://twitter.com/niadla (@niadla) and is keen that all people with an interest in mental health engage together as a community to support good practice and challenge discrimination. She has teaching and research interests in women's health, physical and mental health, social media and health education.

Katie Letchfield is a qualified occupational therapist currently working for a Mental Health Trust in London, UK. Her first degree was in economics and sociology from Manchester University. Katie has worked in the third sector for a social enterprise to engage young disadvantaged people in the construction industry. Katie has a particular interest in older people and is passionate about all things Spanish.

Ellouise Long graduated from Middlesex in 2012 with a BA in Sociology with Psychology and then in 2014 completed the MSc Psychology (Conversion). Ellouise has been involved in a number of projects such as the EU funded 'Developing Research Informed Good Practice Policing and Industry Collaborative Models in Preventing Online Child Abuse and

Profiling Child Victims' project with CATs and is also employed in the Psychology department at Middlesex University as a Senior Graduate Academic Assistant. Her MPhil/PhD is focusing on online behaviour and, in particular, internet trolling. The overall aim of her doctoral research therefore is to attempt to provide a relevant and adequate typology of trolling behaviour online. Other aspects of her research include attempting to provide a clear definition of the phenomenon and to look in more depth at explanations for trolling. Ellouise is also involved in the Forensic Psychology Research Group based at Middlesex University.

Mary Martin retired in 2014 after 40 years teaching English at secondary schools in Cambridge. She was head of teacher training as well as deputy principal, with responsibilities for promoting evidence based teaching via research with all staff and supporting training teachers on their University of Cambridge Master's Programmes. Her research interests include investigating the impact of thinking skills in cross curricular literacy, the impact of gender in developing oracy and literacy in single sex and mixed classes and an exploration into the role of dialogue and restorative justice processes in improving attitudes to diversity. Through her interest in equal opportunities she developed the PEOPLE people programme (Pupils' Equal Opportunities Policy Means Learning for Everyone). This comprised strategies for working with pupils to raise awareness of and build a culture of understanding in order to implement conflict resolution leading to greater tolerance and respect for the individual spanning all aspects of diversity. For more information and resources on PEOPLE people visit peoplepeoplemovement.wordpress.com.

Alfonso Pezzella is an Associate Lecturer in Mental Health at Middlesex University London. Alfonso holds a BSc (Hons) in Psychology and an MSc in Applied Clinical Health Psychology. Alfonso teaches on a variety of topics including research methods to social work students, SPSS workshops, mental health, LGB&T issues and transcultural issues in health. Alfonso's research includes working on large scale European projects with other European countries. He has a strong interest in mental health and LGB&T research and has also worked on various research projects on LGB&T inclusion in the curriculum in health and social care education, coming out in the workplace and LGB&T and mental health. Alfonso has authored several papers and research reports specialising in nursing education, mental health and LGB&T issues in health and social care. Alfonso has a professional Twitter feed @AlfPezzella where he enjoys bringing the community together and discussing topics regarding mental health, LGB&T, psychology and education.

Jennifer Power is a Senior Research Fellow at the Australian Research Centre in Sex, Health and Society at La Trobe University in Melbourne. Her work is focused on sexuality, sexual health and HIV. She has a PhD and is published widely on topics related to parenting and reproductive choices among lesbian, gay, bisexual and transgender communities. Her research on HIV is about people's experiences living with HIV and community activism in response to HIV.

Damien W. Riggs is an Associate Professor in social work at Flinders University, Australia and an Australian Research Council Future Fellow. He is the author of over 200 publications in the fields of gender, family, and mental health, including (with Clare Bartholomaeus) Transgender people and education (Palgrave, 2018) and (with Clemence Due) A critical approach to surrogacy: Reproductive desires and demands (Routledge, 2017). He is a Fellow of the Australian Psychological Society and a psychotherapist who specialises in working with young transgender people.

Peter Ryan is Emeritus Professor of Mental Health at Middlesex University and has conducted a wide range of large European studies on user involvement, parental mental health and homophobic and transphobic bullying. Recent projects include working with the World Health Organisation to improve the knowledge and skills of professionals in Turkey who are responsible for training in mental health and a mixed method study of Disability employment in the NHS. Peter has a background in social work.

Annie Pullen Sansfaçon is a Social Worker and an Associate Professor at the University of Montreal's School of social work. She has a PhD in Ethics, Social Work from De Montfort University, UK. Her work focuses on the development of anti-oppressive theories, approaches and methodologies to promote ethical and emancipatory practice in social work. She has extensive experience in Social Action Research, a form of Community Based Participatory Action Research, and in Self-Directed Groupwork, a method of intervention to work with oppressed groups, based on the same principles. She is the principal investigator of two funded projects aimed at better understanding the experiences of trans children and their families (CIRH 2016–2019; SSRCH 2016–2019) and is one of the co-founders and current Vice-President of Gender Creative Kids Canada, a Montreal-based community organisation working with trans children and youth and their families. She is also a researcher at the Research Institute for Public Health of the University of Montreal, a member of the Quebec Research Chair on Homophobia and an Associate Researcher at the School of Social Work of the University of Stellenbosch, in South Africa.

Rachael M. Scicluna is a Lecturer at the School of Anthropology and Conservation at The University of Kent, UK, and a Research Affiliate within the Mediterranean Institute at the University of Malta. She is the author of Home and Sexuality: The 'Other' Side of the Kitchen (2017), an ethnography that explores the domestic lives of older lesbian feminists in

London. Rachael is also Co-Director of the Home and Research Network based at the University of Kent. Her research interests are queer anthropology, kinship and family formations, gender identity, sexuality, politics and home in England and South Europe.

Rosalind Scott is a Science Teacher and has taught in secondary schools across UK and Southern Africa. She became an Advanced Skills teacher of science and began coaching teachers before taking a leading role promoting partnership in Clacton and Harwich Education Action Zone. As Director of Tilbury and Chadwell Excellence Cluster her remit included teacher development, setting up Inclusion Centres to ensure that no child was excluded from school and working with gifted and talented children. At Voyager Academy, Comberton Academy Trust, Rosalind was assistant head with responsibility for behaviour and inclusion; she became Director of Partnership involved in developing peer review in the Schools Partnership Programme. Rosalind continues to work in Leadership Development and Organisational Analysis and is a local councillor.

Paul Simpson is a Senior Lecturer in applied health and social care at Edge Hill University, UK. As a sociologist, he is the Principal Investigator of cross-disciplinary research initiative, Older People's Understandings of Sexuality (OPUS) and has published extensively on various aspects of ageing sexuality and masculinities.

1 Sexuality, sexual and gender identities and intimacy research in social work and social care

What does the life course lens have to offer?

Trish Hafford-Letchfield and
Priscilla Dunk-West

Introduction

This introductory chapter sets out the context for addressing new areas of scholarship in sexuality and gender identities and the significance of including the voices of LGBT populations in social work scholarship. These impact well-being, but are not at the forefront of social work education and practice. The overall book content is linked to our examination of the life course in social work which can otherwise be institutionalised in their approach and themes. The chapter synopses are provided and broader public health and well-being themes are highlighted from their content. The chapter calls for readers to challenge normative life course theories so as to promote human rights and justice for marginalised individuals and groups.

This book follows on from the success of *Sexuality and Sexual Identities in Social Work: Research and Reflections from Women in the Field* (Dunk-West & Hafford-Letchfield, 2011), which brought together contemporary research about sexualities by women researchers. This second edited collection aims to compliment, enrich and extend social work knowledge of sexuality, sexual identity and intimacy for those working in the caring professions. Whereas *Sexuality and Sexual Identities* outlined relevant research from women's perspectives, this collection includes relevant new areas of scholarship in sexuality including trans perspectives, masculinities and the voices of LGBT populations during life course trajectories and settings that impact on well-being but are not at the forefront of practice. Traditional texts on the life course used within professional education and practice are to some degree institutionalised in their approach and themes. This book, however, draws on empirical research which picks up on the broader public health and well-being agenda with a strong focus on challenging normative theories so as to promote human rights and justice for marginalised individuals and groups.

In this sense, the new collection opens up new possibilities for better understanding sexuality in social work: something which is needed despite some shifts in understanding this field since our first publication in 2011. This edited collection therefore contains relevant empirical work and theorising about sexuality, intimacy and gender not currently found in a traditional course on life course theory and practice.

This book examines the relationship between sexuality, sexual identities and intimacies and the life course and showcases a range of issues pertinent to social work through these particular lenses. The reason that a 'life course' perspective is important to this text is because of the need to tie together the varying 'strands' of sexuality. In social work, sexuality is a growing area of scholarly inquiry. Given the role that intimate relationships play in social and individual lives, much more needs to be achieved in order to value this area of scholarship. For example, social work's relationship with sexuality, normally positioned and categorised through concepts of anti-discriminatory and anti-oppressive theories, is yet to be fulling integrated into social work curricula.

In this chapter, we provide an orientation to the subject matter contained in this edited collection and we begin to explore some of the concepts central to the themes in this book. First, it is important to outline the reason for the arrangement of the chapters: thus, we now consider what role the life course approach plays in such an arrangement.

The life course approach

We know from both sociology (Hunt, 2016) and psychology (Elder, 1998) that questions and expressions of identity are pertinent throughout the life course. One of the benefits of a life course perspective is that it accounts for social, historical and biographical contexts in theorising about life stages (Elder, 1998). A life course approach sees life from beginning to end: birth to death. In social work, developmental theories not only inform childhood, but apply across the life span. Informed by theorists such as Erikson (1950, 1968), such a lens views age as bringing about a particular 'stage' tied up with identity. If we consider the role of intimacy, relationships, families, sexual and gender identities across the life course and in relation to social expectations and biographical events, we can begin to see that these issues are manifest throughout the life span in particular iterations. For example, from birth, the notion of family, being parented and the learning of social relationships occurs (Mead, 1913).

Sexualities and beyond

Up until now, sexuality has been treated as a specialist topic or area of practice whereas we contend that issues to do with sexual and gender identity cut across all areas of social work, and to relegate it to any specialist topic, stage of the life course or single field of practice would be very misleading. Sexuality is an umbrella term that relates to the private dimension in which people live out their sexual, intimate and/or emotional desires. Sexual identity, on the other hand, suggests a stance in orientation, it provokes categorical discernment. Thus, sexual and gender identities relate to defining the nature of one's attractions and desires, gendered relationships and include terms that pronounce this, including lesbian, gay, bisexual, queer, heterosexual, cis, questioning and many others. There are also broader terms which relate to sexuality and gender. Intimacy, friendships and relationships are examples that are explored in this edited collection. The term intimacy can be associated with sexual relationships as well as used to describe the closeness inherent to non-sexual relationships. The fact that this term has evolved to include the latter speaks to the shifting nature of theorising brought about through historical, social and political movements. Thus:

> Over the course of modernity, various discourses of intimacy have evolved to designate types of relationship that the modern subject [implicitly male, white, heterosexual, bourgeois, reproductive] might establish with a variety of others. 'Traditional' discourses of intimacy have referred to physical contact, sex, romance or passionate love, invariably with a spouse. Newer discourse of intimacy have emerged that refer to the non-sexual relationships of family life.
>
> (Attwood, Hakim, & Winch, 2017, p. 249)

Two points emerge from this quote that are relevant to our project. First, in this edited collection, this newer concept of intimacy is explored in relation to the role that others play in people's lives. Second, individual conceptualisations of intimacy and sexuality must be seen in their broader social contexts. Thus, though sexuality and gender are often conceptualised as 'private' and merely individually experienced, they occur in social and historical contexts (Dunk-West, 2012). Tackling social injustice is at the core of social work. Inequality, trans-, bi- and homophobia are enduring issues for people who identify outside dominant heteronormative and rigid gender discourses, and these too ought to be of interest to the discipline of social work and are therefore examined in this book. Since social work's core purpose is to work with individuals across the life course, issues relevant to relationships, gender and sexual identities and inequalities are crucial areas which need to be better understood. This edited collection therefore showcases the very latest theorising and research in these areas. At the end of each chapter we have ensured that the empirical work upon which each chapter is based is translated into recommendations for social work practice. The key messages for practice section therefore concludes each chapter and are included to assist the social work student, practitioner or academic reading this collection. We now move on to a summary of the chapters contained in this edited book.

Chapter synopses

In Chapter 2, Annie Pullen-Sansfaçon reviews the evidence on a neglected section of the population, that of gender non-conforming children and trans youth. Being able to respond and support these children and young people is of growing significance, yet the underpinning evidence is still lacking in many areas and what does exist has many gaps to help our understanding. Strong evidence on the degree of violence, discrimination, poor mental health and high-risk factors for health provide strong indications for preventative work in social work practice. Pullen-Sansfaçon also highlights the stress on families, parents and carers who need quality information, guidance and support to be able to access the best care for their children, and who also face stigma and poor-quality services. She highlights how important it is for social work to engage holistically and strategically as well as to support the individuals and families involved. As we will see in the chapter on homophobic and transphobic bullying, being a partner with local communities through schools, local health providers and other stakeholders is essential to challenge discrimination and oppression and to advocate on behalf of marginalised populations.

Chapter 3 looks at homophobic and transphobic bullying in schools and draws on findings from the European research project RAINBOW-HAS (Rights through alliances: Innovating and networking both within homes and schools'). Partners from the UK (Trish Hafford-Letchfield, Christine Cocker, Peter Ryan, Mary Martin, Rosalind Scott, and Sarah Carr) highlight some of the key findings from RAINBOW-HAS and enable us to get a good sense of where homophobic and transphobic bullying in the UK is situated in terms of the education policy literature. They use this review to foreground a case study which engaged with two secondary schools to develop and pilot a family and student led intervention aimed at preventing homophobic and transphobic bullying. Given the tendency for silence on LGBT issues more broadly, this practice example encourages readers to reflect on how they position themselves in relation to working with young people from the LGBT community and how they might take account of bullying experiences, targeted violence and hostility that young people may experience as a result of their sexual and gender identities. Using a community based intervention which engages with young people, their families and education provides a practice example for how collaboration can be more active in their contribution to young people's well-being in education through LGBT rights-based advocacy.

In Chapter 4, continuing with themes associated with earlier life, Katie Letchfield and Trish Hafford-Letchfield invite us to think outside the box in their report of a research study into friendship and intimacy in young women. The phenomenon of friendship and its function and purpose within social work and social care is significantly under-researched and so this chapter attempts to do this through a sociological analysis of the function of symbols and ritual in relation to ideals of 'friendships' among young women. It draws principally from a small qualitative study involving semi-structured interviews with five women aged 18–25 years during which they discussed their friendships. Letchfield and Hafford-Letchfield draw out the importance of intimacy in friendships for young women within this stage of the life course from the key themes emerging from their data. Their research focused particularly on the role of gender specific symbols and ritual, how these relate to gender roles in young women and the significance of external influences on their friendship practices. The findings indicated that not only do rituals and symbols create and support internal intimacy, but also constitute practices informed by a cultural ideal of what it means to be a 'friend'. This suggests very unique implications for how social work assessment and interventions takes these into account when working with young people and other service user groups. It is important to be aware of relationships beyond the traditional family or network commonly conceptualised with social work assessment and care support. There are important messages about how social workers value social relationships beyond the family and their functions in providing support for expressions of intimacy, agency and identities in young women. Further, conceptualising friendships highlights the ways that friendship experience is shaped by minority status and inequalities and the support needed to develop cross group friendships which promote cultural competence or dialogue between different social groups and reinforce young people's own identities through the life course.

Moving to consider mid-life course issues, in Chapter 5 Paul Simpson also explores friendships, this time in a midlife context. He explores a very much neglected topic by examining the means through which middle-aged and older gay men differentiate themselves from forms of intimacy and relating associated with heterosexual people. Writing from the UK, Paul draws on in-depth interviews with 27 middle-aged gay men living in Manchester and develops themes on 'friendship families', a concept which has been developed by other LGBT scholars. He argues that two major shifts occur in midlife away from the biological/biolegal family of origin and the Manchester 'gay village'/'commercial scene' towards domestically staged 'friendship family'. The latter represents a creative extension of the gay scene/kinship. Such family helps maintain a sense of identity, self-worth and inclusion in one aspect of gay culture. It was narrated as a space that helped men to develop the 'ageing capital' – the age-inflected emotional, cognitive and political resources to withstand/contest homophobia and gay ageism. In this research project, subjects also used the 'resources of ageing' (Heaphy, 2007) to question heteronormative notions of family and practice non-monogamy. However, whilst men's experiences of homes and neighbourhoods were generally affirmative, representation of home(s) as empowering space(s) is complicated and undermined for various reasons. Whilst some informants experienced disadvantaged access to or exclusion from friendship family for socio-economic and cultural reasons (often connected with homophobia), gay ageism online and (ageist) homophobia in neighbourhoods can render the home a site of risk, compromising its status as space of freedom, self-expression and physical and emotional safety.

Simpson draws attention to the value of friendship family as a way of distinguishing and framing middle-aged gay men's relational experiences. For social workers, it is important to recognise and value this form of kinship which does important political and emotional work in empowering middle-aged gay men living in large cities and who may not be able to rely on their family of origin (or younger gay men) for support. Simpson illustrates how friendship family is characterised by an ethic of care and mutual understanding that enables middle-aged gay to men express their 'authentic' ageing selves freed from the ageist gaze that dominates experiences of the gay commercial scene. Social workers need to take note of this critical space in which to develop the resources of ageing capital and technologies of the self to contest homophobia, gay ageism and to resist pressures towards monogamy and thus assert the value of alternative ways of relating.

Chapter 6 returns to the topic of life course issues with people with transgender identities and how transgender people negotiate intimate relationships. In this chapter, Damien Riggs, Henry von Doussa and Jennifer Power remind us of the important relationship between discrimination and poor mental health in transgender populations and the importance of research for documenting these experiences of marginalisation and victimisation, and for identifying the needs of transgender people in terms of mental health service provisions. However, this chapter also contributes to a consistently overlooked aspect of the lives of transgender people in relation to their experiences of negotiating intimate relationships. They provide an important overview of previous literature on the topic of transgender people and intimate relationships, before reporting on findings from their own Australian qualitative study. Importantly, the findings suggest both that understanding transgender people's experiences of intimacy cannot occur absent of an understanding of the effects of discrimination, and that recognising the impact of discrimination does not explain all there is to know about transgender people's experiences of intimacy. Beyond the impact of both discrimination and cisgenderism, for many transgender people experiences of intimacy are fulfilling and meaningful. Riggs, Von Dousa and Power help us to understand that those who work with transgender clients must be mindful of the importance of engaging with transgender people's experiences of intimacy and the dangers of taking a developmentally normative approach. They encourage us to incorporate a positive focus on intimacy when working with transgender people so as to support their future vision of living fulfilling and meaningful intimate lives as they determine them to be.

Chapter 7 looks at the issue of employment which for many people can be a significant activity for up to half of their life course, and with increasing longevity and demography, is likely to continue to be an important space in which we interact and contribute to society. Alfonso Pezzella examines the impact of institutionalised heteronormativity on LGBT employee's relationships at work and focuses on the issue of disclosure of sexual identity and orientation, commonly known as 'coming out'. Despite legislative gains on equality and rights in the workplace in many developing countries, the choice to disclose one's sexual identity in every social role in the workplace is still controversial and sensitive for many LGBTQ individuals. This may involve them weighing up the risk of coming out to their colleagues and employer which in turn has the potential to impact on their professional career and prospects, as well as expose them to discrimination, harassment and oppression (Hafford-Letchfield, 2012). Drawing on a local case study in one university, Pezzella explores factors in a typical heteronormative institution which influence LGBT employee's expression of identities, well-being, career choices and decision making. He uses these findings to help us think about our own institutional environments and specifically some of the knowledge, skills and awareness needed for ensuring inclusive support for employees in care settings so that we are enable and respect diversity of those providing as well as using services. There are also important messages for what we include in our curriculum and practice education and how we support learning about and with LGBT communities.

Social work is all about relationships, and Chapter 8 examines the utility of knowledge about relationship quality for practice. Jill M. Chonody, Jacqui Gabb, Mike Killian and Priscilla Dunk-West share their international study into long-term relationships to examine the notion of relationship quality in intimate coupling. Relationship quality is a concept which is potentially fraught with assumptions and cannot be understood without reference to broader social issues and conditions which shape intimate coupling in the contemporary world. Chonody, Gabb, Killian and Dunk-West challenge the questions we ask and the epistemological positions we take up when assessing relationships, all of which position relationship quality normatively. The authors draw on findings from a mixed methods research study, 'Enduring Love: couple relationships in the 21st century', and a combined data set, drawn primarily from the UK, USA and Australia. They encourage a strengths-based approach to the measurement of relationship quality by focusing on positive elements of the relationship instead of a problems-focused agenda. This has the capacity to extend understandings of how relationship quality is manifest, in an everyday sense, and to enrich knowledge on what constitutes relationship quality in a working relationship. As such, it has the potential to make a significant contribution to and have practical applications in the fields of relationship support and intervention which is the bread and butter of social work.

Chapter 9 takes us into an examination of the concept of bisexuality – a topic hardly discussed within the social work literature and arguably one of the most invisible categories used in the LGBT acronym. This invisibility and lack of recognition of the needs of bisexuals across the life course is important to address in the practice of social workers and illustrative of the complex and changing relationships between sexuality and sexual identities which need to become more visible if we are to use the bisexual label authentically. Kathryn Almack, Rebecca Jones and Rachael Scicluna help us to appreciate the key role that social work has to play in tackling inequalities and their impact in people's lives given the recent empirical evidence on bisexual citizen's vulnerability to poverty and poor mental health. The chapter discusses both theoretical and empirical research on bisexuality, particularly illustrated through three case studies discussion of selected case studies from their own research to further examine key issues in applying research into practice for social workers. Their case studies illustrate ways in which an accumulation of a lifetime of experiences of bisexual people or bisexual relationship histories can lead to what (the editors of this book) identify as 'institutionalised harms', which may be individual, organisational and structural. In turn, there are profound impacts and implications on individual requirements for support, perceptions of support available from social work services, as well as concerns in approaching services possibly due to past discriminatory experiences for bisexual people.

The final part of the book starts to look at later life, or ageing studies as it is sometimes known. Both Chapters 10 and 11 focus on aspects of women's ageing. Chapter 10 presents findings from a quantitative study on older women living alone. Hafiz T.A. Khan, Nicky Lambert and Trish Hafford-Letchfield look at some of the factors associated with health and well-being of women living alone in later life using data collected in the 'Understanding Society' 2012; a nationwide longitudinal survey that captures important information on the life course trajectories of individuals in the UK. By looking at variables associated with health and well-being, they identify important determinants when looking at the increasing prevalence of women living alone. Within the increasing trend of women living alone over time and space, there is a need to adapt and develop more accurate measures and research designs in order to begin to understand the factors impacting the nature of ageing for those who are living alone. The importance of comparing profiles for different groups of older women is noted in order to consider the development of research priorities which support inclusive positive ageing. Household status and living arrangements are important for individuals to satisfy several goals, for example, privacy, companionship and care, socio-psychological needs such as by staying connected as well as for practical reasons as in making domestic arrangements and economies of scale. For those of us working in care services, we need to be aware of the potential for how living alone lowers the levels of social and familial support in later life, and not only the risk of having insufficient support, but the potential loss of quality in relationships including sexuality and intimacy.

Chapter 11 presents stories of intimacy and sexuality in later life from a marginalised group of the population, who are ageing without a partner or children. Nicky Lambert, Trish Hafford-Letchfield, Hafiz T.A. Khan, Ellouise Long, Dominique Brady and Lisa Clarke present selected findings from a study on what they term as 'solo' women and reflect on this group within the context of the impact of the rise in non-traditional family relationships on successful ageing. There has been limited research that seeks to understand these women's support networks, social connectedness and personal relationships. Their chapter draws on selected findings from a study which has investigated some of the dynamics and issues impacting solo women in later life using a range of methods including a literature review, demographic analysis, an online survey and interview data. Drawing on some of the qualitative data, they provide a snapshot of solo women's own subjective perspectives about the links between their relationship status and well-being in later life, particularly in relation to sexuality and intimacy. Social workers tend not to consider intimate relationships in terms of their contribution to well-being such as physical, emotional and psychological health and how these are conceptualised in care settings. The findings from the solo study is discussed in the context of this wider picture and Lambert et al. conclude with recommendations for practitioners in relation to how we encourage and facilitate the voices of solo women in order to design and provide tailored support to meet their unique needs.

In the final chapter, Chapter 12, we return to the key issues inherent to this book and argue that social work education about intimacy, relationships, sexualities and gender equips social workers with the skills necessary to work with their clients. The editors use this final chapter to synthesise the findings of the studies contained in this book and make suggestions about how such findings might be utilised to be of benefit to the people with whom we work.

We hope you enjoy this second collection of research on sexuality and intimacy and hope that you find it as interesting as we did in editing it.

References

Attwood, F., Hakim, J., & Winch, A. (2017). Mediated intimacies: Bodies, technologies and relationships. *Journal of Gender Studies, 26*(3), 249–253.

Dunk-West. (2012). The sexual self and social work and policy, or, why teenage pregnancy prevention programmes miss the point. *Social Work & Society, 10*(2), 1–3.

Dunk-West, P., & Hafford-Letchfield, T. (Eds.). (2011). *Sexual identities and sexuality in social work: Research and reflections from women in the field.* Surrey, UK: Ashgate.

Elder, G. H. (1998). The life course as developmental theory. *Child Development*, 69(1), 1–12.

Erikson, E. H. (1950). *Childhood and society*. New York, NY: W. W. Norton & Co. Inc.

Erikson, E. H. (1968). *Identity, youth and crisis*. New York, NY: W. W. Norton.

Hunt, S. (2016). *The life course: A sociological introduction* (2nd ed.). London, UK: Palgrave.

Mead, G. H. (1913). The social self. In F. C. Silva (Ed.), *G.H. Mead: A Reader*. Abingdon, UK: Routledge.

2 Gender non-conforming children, trans youth and their family

Identifying best evidences and practices for social work interventions

Annie Pullen Sansfaçon

Introduction

Gender non-conforming children and trans youth are a segment of the population with an increasingly high profile in public discourse but whose needs remain largely misunderstood and neglected. For the purpose of this chapter, this group includes children and young people aged 25 and younger who do not identify with the gender they were assigned at birth, the sex registered on their birth certificate. While research is starting to emerge on this topic, it remains scarce and piecemeal, especially research publications concerning prepubertal trans children. However, empirical information currently available, as well as best practice guidelines produced by professional organisations, point towards types of interventions and involvement that can best help social work support trans youth and their families. This chapter reviews current knowledge on gender non-conforming children, trans youth and their experience, and explores some of the resilience and vulnerability factors that recent research has identified. It also describes the experience of families who have a trans child. Last, based on this cumulated evidence and available practice guidelines, the chapter discusses the most promising way to interact with this population segment, from a social work perspective.

Trans youth is an umbrella term that may include gender non-conforming and trans children and youth, a group that is heterogonous in its composition. "Trans youth" may claim for themselves, or may be given/imposed identity markers such as transsexual, transgender, gender non-conforming, gender-queer, gender variant, gender creative or others. Some of these young people may feel strongly that they identify with "male" or "female", while others may adopt gender-fluid or non-binary identification markers. Some may or may not, currently or in the future, pursue different forms and pathways of transitions. These can be described as "social transition" (i.e. adopting a gender-affirming name and pronoun, presenting oneself in gender-concordant clothing), "medical transition" (i.e. puberty blockers and hormone replacement therapy (HRT) or surgical procedures) and "legal transition" (i.e. legal name and gender-marker change where it is allowed). Those who may not pursue such transitions may do so out of choice or as a result of barriers to access (family, school, the community at large or the impossibility to do so because of legal obstacles, for example). What this otherwise diverse population of youth has in common, however, is that they face disproportional levels of adversity and an uneven distribution of life chances. This is in spite of recent social and legal gains in some states and jurisdictions in the recognition, acceptance, and celebration of gender and sexual diversity in society.

Identifying the trans population and their needs

Knowledge on the topic is growing but still sketchy. Whereas quantitative research has shed some light on some of the experiences of transgender children and youth (See for example, Clark et al. 2014; Olson et al. 2016), it still stops short of providing an in-depth understanding of the reality. Publications also generally discuss medical transition and psycho-social treatment (for example, De Vries and Cohen-Kettenis 2012; Mallon 2009; Olson, Forbes, and Belzer 2011).

Furthermore, little insight into the lives of gender non-conforming/trans children is currently available. Most research in the field tends to discuss transgender prepubertal children and postpubertal youth together, and little evidence focuses specifically on gender non-conforming and trans children before the onset of puberty. In general, many questions remain unanswered in the literature on the topic (Drescher and Byne 2012), such as the percentage of transgender children globally, or how many gender non-conforming children identify as trans adults later in life. When attempting to provide answers to those questions, publications seem to highlight significantly differing statistics and figures (De Vries and Cohen-Kettenis 2012; Pyne 2014).

Aside from helping to assess plans for which services to provide, some wonder whether such statistics are useful, or even possible to obtain and confirm, since what constitutes gender conformity is intimately related to cultural practice and therefore varies among societies (Pyne 2014). What is considered a gender non-conforming youth may differ from one culture to another; it may also be difficult to know exactly how many trans children and youth there are because many young people do not affirm their true gender identity until much later, if at all, because of the hostile context in which they grow up. Furthermore, despite increased visibility in the media, transgender children and youth often remain invisible (Hellen 2009), because their gender expression may be inhibited by parental and social pressures that force them to conform with the gender norms that are defined by the majority. As a participant in a recent Quebec research study said: "Gender non-conforming kids are like baby pigeons. They are around, but no one seems to be noticing them" (cited in Pullen Sansfaçon, Robichaud, and Dumais-Michaud 2015: 50).

Yet, gender identity development seems to happen in a majority of cases before adulthood (Beemyn and Rankin 2011; Olson, Forbes, and Belzer 2011), as early as 3 or 4 years old (Ehrensaft 2014a). A youth's sense of incongruence between gender identity and gender assigned at birth would be felt around 10.4 years of age, with trans self-identification around 14.3 years and coming out to others around 14.5 years of age (Grossman and D'Augelli 2006).

More recently, two significant research publications have contributed to deepen understandings of gender identity development specifically in transgender children (Olson et al. 2015, 2016). Notably, Olson et al. (2015) examined the feeling of gender identity in 23 transgender children aged between 5 and 12 years who were supported by their parents, compared it to 18 cisgender children (their siblings) and 32 cisgender control participants of the same age, and concluded that:

> On both more-controllable self-report measures and less-controllable implicit measures, our group of transgender children showed a clear indication that they thought of themselves in terms of their expressed gender. Their responses were indistinguishable from those of the two cisgender control groups, when matched by gender identity. They showed a clear preference for peers and objects endorsed by peers who shared their expressed gender, an explicit and implicit identity that aligned with their expressed gender, and a strong implicit preference for their expressed gender.
>
> (Olson et al. 2015: 7)

In other words, this empirical evidence underscores that the feeling of gender identity felt by transgender children is no different from the feeling of gender identity felt by the two other groups of non-transgender participants.

The experience of trans children and youth

The current body of knowledge suggests that this group is especially vulnerable to abuse and violence (Nuttbrock et al. 2010, 2012; Roberts et al. 2012), including cyber-intimidation and bullying (Blumenfeld and Cooper 2010), and is over-represented in rates of homelessness (Cochran 2002; Crossley 2015; Sifra Quintana, Rosenthal, and Krehely 2010) and of arrest, detention, and incarceration (Garnette et al. 2011). They are at high risk for use and misuse of alcohol and other substances (Newcomb, Heinz, and Mustanski 2012) are more likely to engage in risky sexual practices, and to rely on survival sex for housing or sex work as a source of income, in particular when they are homeless (Walls and Bell 2011); they are at high risk of HIV infection (Brennan et al. 2012; Wilson et al. 2012), and finally, they exhibit high rates of mental health issues (Menvielle 2012), suicide attempts and suicide (Liu and Mustanski 2012; Mustanski and Lui 2012). Indeed, according to a recent study in the province of Ontario (Canada) on trans persons of all ages (*n* = 433), 77% reported having seriously considered suicide at one point in their lives, while 43% reported having attempted suicide (Bauer et al. 2013). Of this 43%, 78% were under the age of 24 at the time of their first attempt and 36% under the age of 15 (Bauer et al. 2013).

But experiences may differ greatly, depending on the support they receive and the environment in which young people grow up. Various sources of acceptance and support are identified as factors that contribute positively to trans youth's well-being beyond aspects related to medical transition, while rejection, stigmatisation and abuse negatively affect youth's mental and physical development and health (Hegarty 2009). Moreover, lack of parental support and familial abuse have both been identified as key factors increasing the likelihood of experiencing homelessness (Durso and Gates 2012). Inversely, parental acceptance and larger familial support, in both the private and public spheres (Ajeto 2009), are key factors associated with trans youth's positive life experiences (Brill and Peper 2013). On that score, Travers et al. (2012: 3) discovered that "the impact of strong parental support can be clearly seen in the 93% reduction in reported suicide attempts for youth who indicated their parents were strongly supportive of their gender identity and gender expression. Another recent study undertaken with 73 transgender children aged 3–12 as well as two control groups (sibling and general population) of similar age, found that the mental health of transgender children supported by their parents was not significantly different from their cisgender (non-transgender) counterpart with regard to depression, and that only a small difference could be observed with regard to anxiety (Olson et al. 2016). Therefore, it would appear that affirming the true gender identity of children and offering them strong support may lead to more positive outcomes for this group of young people.

Furthermore, schools have been shown to play an important role in the integration and support, or in the rejection and alienation, of trans youth (Wyss 2004). Other contexts where integration and support or rejection and stigmatisation can take place are religious institutions (Glenn 2000), ethno-cultural communities (Bith-Melander et al. 2010; Saketopoulou 2011), health-care and social services agencies (Burgess 2000; Price Minter 2012; Singh 2012; Stieglitz 2010), LGBT community organisations and support groups and the job market (Singh, Meng, and Hansen 2014). General social connectedness beyond familial support (DiFulvio 2011), online interactions with peers and access to educational materials (DeHaan et al. 2013; Magee et al. 2012), as well as healthy romantic relationships (Bauermeister et al. 2010) can also positively impact trans youth's resilience. However, if individual elements such as psychological resilience may affect youth's coping abilities in the face of violence (Grossman, D'Augelli, and Frank 2011), the impact of psychological and physical gender-based abuse on trans individuals' experiences of major depression, suicidality (Nuttbrock et al. 2010) and post-traumatic stress disorder (Roberts et al. 2012) remains considerable.

To summarise, gender identity develops quite early on in the lives of young people and existing research points to a variety of sources (abuse, parental support, school integration, access to care, etc.) in young persons' lives that can either act as positive or negative influences on their well-being. However, parental support and broader community support, such as that provided by schools, seems to be the most promising path to insuring better mental health outcomes for those youth. Since parental support seems to be essential to trans youth's thriving, we will now turn to exploring parents' and caregivers' experience in supporting their offspring, so that social work involvement can start to work with systems as well as with individuals.

Parents and caregivers of gender non-conforming and trans youth

Acceptance of a transgender child may be an important challenge for many families. Indeed, accepting the idea that a child may affirm a different gen-der than the one the parents have always known often comes as a shock (Pullen Sansfaçon et al. 2015). While this may take time, obtaining a for-mal diagnosis of gender variance seems to help parents to accept their child generally (Riggs and Due 2015). This was echoed in Pullen Sansfaçon et al. (2015) research with parents who, while discussing labels used to described their child's gender identity, asserted that labels and diagnoses such as that of gender variance were sometimes helpful because they were better known by the public. Participants added that it provided some sort of outside vali-dation and recognition of their children's experience.

Once the parents begin to accept the child's gender identity, they can start supporting him or her, but further barriers may crop up, as some report experiencing isolation and rejection from extended family and the commu-nity at large (Pullen Sansfaçon 2015). Challenges may also arise for families when negotiating with institutions such as schools and civic, religious or sport associations (Meadow 2011).

For example, emerging conflict between parents is a potential challenge faced by families who support a trans child (Pullen Sansfaçon et al. 2015); in addition, research has found that fathers tend to have more difficulty ac-cepting their child than mothers (Riggs and Due 2015). Anecdotal evidence show that it is not infrequent that parents quarrel about the best way to parent a gender non-conforming child or a trans youth, some even requiring a court judgment, as in the case of one family that disagreed on the care of their transgender child (Canadian Press 2016).

Not surprisingly, parents who support their children also tend to expe-rience anxiety and social isolation. Those with younger children who have to provide their consent to access services, for example, may feel anxious when making their decision, worried that the child will blame them later on (for example, allowing the child to take a medication that blocks their hormones before they can themselves consent to such care, or supporting social transition at school or in the community) (Pullen Sansfaçon et al. 2015). Parents also feel anxious, as they feel some of the struggles their children may themselves face. As Ehrensaft (2011: 213) explains,

> the specter of violence or even death may become either a loud siren or a lurking shadow that can render clear thinking very difficult. And the anxiety about danger and negativity from the outside world can get all mixed up with the parents' own internal doubt or gender ghosts from the past, creating a rather noxious emotional potion. This angst is hard to escape and should be held in mind by any mental health professionals working with parents, with the aim of helping them embrace and protect their gender creative child.
>
> (213)

The multiple possible challenges that may face trans youth, as summarised earlier in this chapter, seem to be a concern for many of their parents/carers, thus leading to increased anxiety about their child's well-being. Parents who experience this anxiety on a daily basis do so, more often than not, without formal networks of support (Riley et al. 2011). Indeed, services for parents themselves are scarce, a situation that contributes further to their experience of stress and anxiety (Pullen Sansfaçon et al. 2015). In fact, access to specialist care, either for their children or for themselves (helping them to cope with the situation) is limited (Riley et al. 2013). For example, Pullen Sansfaçon et al. (2015) in her Montreal-based research documented how specialist services are not always available, and finding an appropriate clinician to work with their child can be difficult.

In addition to the challenge of finding specialised care, access to general services can also be difficult, especially where it is not possible to access identification documents that match the gender identity of the child. This issue is not specific to transgender children and youth. It also applies to transgender adults, and may lead to further challenges, such as when a parent is accessing general services with their child. Parents are put in a position where they need to explain countless times that their child is transgender, often in places where confidentiality cannot be guaranteed (such as at a registration desk for example).

Research into access to services for transgender adults has reported many issues that are also experienced by young people. For example, Stroumsa (2014) explains that hostile environments, lack of knowledge by professionals and stigmatisation and discrimination when accessing services may lead them to avoid those services. These issues can be also faced by parents advocating for their younger children (Grossman and D'Augelli 2006) who cannot themselves access services alone because of their age. In such cases, parents have to negotiate similar situations to those of transgender adults.

It is not surprising to note that the parents are also struggling with access to services as they are often acting as a buffer to some of the experiences faced by trans youth (Pullen Sansfaçon et al. 2014). In fact, parents and allies of transgender children have been found to experience both overt and covert discrimination when accessing services and/or in advocating for their children's needs in the larger community (Cook-Daniels 2011; Pullen Sansfaçon et al. 2015).

To summarise, while the challenges faced by parents are less complex than those faced by trans youth, they nevertheless experience many difficult situations when supporting their children. While emerging evidence stresses that strong parental support is a solid predictor of better mental health outcomes in transgender children and youth (Olson et al. 2015; Travers et al. 2012) and ultimately reduces some of the challenges faced by youth, the support parents provide may not be straightforward, or may not come swiftly when the child affirms his or her gender identity. The final section of this chapter will explore how current knowledge about transgender youth and their families can be used to better inform social-work intervention with this specific segment of the population.

Practicing social work interventions

We have seen thus far that the experience of trans youth is fraught with adversities and as WPATH (2011) underlines, social stigma and discrimination leads to mental health issues and other difficulties, such as rejection from the family or from the broader community (WPATH 2011). Parents can also experience difficulties in accepting and supporting their children.

In preparing to intervene with this specific population, it is important to understand that gender identity should not be pathologised, as the World Professional Association of Transgender Health clearly states:

> the expression of gender characteristics, including identities, that are not stereotypically associated with one's assigned sex at birth is a common and culturally diverse human phenomenon [that] should not be judged as inherently pathological or negative.
>
> (WPATH 2011: 4)

Coherent with this statement, we have also begun to observe, over the past few years, a shift in understanding of gender non-conformity and trans identity among other professional associations. For example, the American Psychiatric Association has undertaken the process of de-pathologising transgender identity with the publication of the Diagnosis and Statistical Manual, version 5 (DSM-V), that now acknowledges that such a diagnosis can have a stigmatising effect on the person and that "gender non-conformity is not itself a mental disorder" (APA 2013: 1). Accordingly, professionals may now diagnose the *consequences* (depression, anxiety, suicidal thoughts, for example) of gender dysphoria, and not the identity itself as it happened in previous version of the DSM. Thus, it is now acknowledged that the difficulty that may emerge from gender dysphoria (the feeling that one's sex assigned at birth does not conform to one's deepest sense of self) may lead to mental health issues, but that gender identity is not the culprit.

Another important step to prepare to intervene with trans youth and their families is to carefully engage in personal introspection and analysis of values, and to identify their own possible bias and discomfort with transgender identities (Ehrensaft 2014b). Since the concept of gender is largely binary, that is male *or* female, in many societies, social workers may well hold negative views about transgender and gender non-conforming people if they have never carefully pondered and educated themselves on the topic. To be well informed about issues faced by transgender children and youth is also considered a core competence of working with this population in social work (Mallon 2009). Without proper introspection and education, social workers may not even realise that the young person in front of them is trying to tell them about their gender identity. Of course, those deeply-held views may naturally lead to act in a way that poses prejudice to the young person by shutting them off or ignoring their request for help.

Furthermore, social workers will have to make choices between different approaches to work with trans youth. Riggs and Due (2015) explain that there are at least two very different approaches that could steer social workers toward very different paths; thus it becomes critical not only to understand the experience of trans youth, but also carefully analyse various approaches and the rationales behind them before intervening.

For example, Riggs and Due (2015) report that some approaches to working with trans youth may consist of helping the parents put limits on the cross-gender behaviour, and that this is particularly helpful when parents have difficulty accepting the transgender child's identity. Zucker et al. (2012: 383), for instance, who advocates this approach, explains that

> if the parents are clear in their desire to have their child feel more comfortable in their own skin, that is, they would like to reduce their child's desire to be of the other gender, the therapeutic approach is organized around this goal.

This approach can seem appealing for some as it may fit better with dominant societal norms which ask boys and girls to adopt mostly stereotypical behaviors and appearance (Riggs and Due 2015). However, while those approaches that are aimed at discouraging or at ignoring gender non-conforming behaviours were once the standard applied when working with children and youth, they are now thought to reinforce gender stereotypical behaviours in gender non-confirming children and youth and have been condemned by a number of scholars and health-care providers because of their negative effects on young people (see for example the Statement on the Affirmation of Gender Diverse Children and Youth). They have also become illegal in some jurisdictions, such as in Ontario, Canada (DiNovo 2015), as well as in a handful of US states. This evolution in the care of transgender youth shows the importance of education, as well as the importance of constantly critically analysing literature on the subject in light of the disciplinary foundations of social work.

Some professional organisations have started to issue guidelines for working with trans youth and gender non-conforming children:

> Gender identity is a core aspect of the self. Any professional's attempt to alter the gender identity or expression of a young person to align with social norms is considered unethical and an abuse of power and authority. Specifically, social workers should reject any attempt to prevent a child from growing up to be transgender, transsexual, two-spirit, gay, lesbian, bisexual or queer.
>
> (Joint Statement by the Canadian Association of
> Social Workers and the Canadian Association
> of Schools of Social Work 2015; 1)

Today, practitioners and scholars increasingly advocate an alternative approach, the *Affirming approach to care* (Bryan 2006; Ehrensaft 2011; Pullen Sansfaçon 2015; Torres Bernal and Coolhart 2012; Wallace and Russell 2013). *Affirming approach to care* is also recognised to be better suited to social work (Mallon 2009). The Affirming approach promotes intervention that considers the person affected the only authority to affirm their gender identity. Accordingly, only the child can know what gender identity they are since the concept of identity, by definition, relates to one's deepest sense of self and is sometimes invisible to others (Poirier et al. 2014).

To do so, Ehrensaft's (2014b) explains that practitioners need to be attuned to what the child is saying, and check for *persistence, insistence, consistence* of the gender identity and the gender expression:

> far from the misperceived instantaneous rubber stamping of gender authenticity based on a child's initial report, the child's discovery of the authentic genderself and the clinician's acknowledgment of that self may move as slow as molasses, and only come months, if not years, after a therapeutic dyad has been firmly in place. So to listen is also to wait.
>
> (Ehrensaft 2014b: 581–82)

The Affirming approach to care fits well with the values of human dignity and self-worth, since it takes into consideration that trans youth should be able to make a decision for themselves about their lives, or in collaboration with their families when they are not legally allowed to provide consent for services. Social workers who work with trans youth and gender non-conforming children should always be guided by the young people and respect their coming-out process, their desire or not to self-disclose their identity and the process and timeline that is most appropriate for them (Poirier et al. 2014: 5). To refuse to acknowledge the child's identity, added to the experience of social rejection, reinforces stigmatisation and may lead to the development of internalised transphobia (Hendricks and Testa (2012) in Testa and Hendrick (2015)), a "discomfort with one's own transgender feelings or identity as a result of internalizing society's normative gender expectations" (WPATH 2011).

But affirming the child's gender identity is only one side of social-work intervention with gender non-conforming children and trans youth. Social workers may also have to support the young person's family to accept the child's gender identity too. In the case of families who do not accept their child, social workers should work with them in the process of acceptance by referring them toward appropriate resources, if necessary, and educating the family about the nature of gender diversity. As families may often be faced with a lack of understanding and acceptance in the broader social environment, social workers should also support families by confronting challenges, such as working with the child and the family to make schools inclusive of all genders, or help civil society recognise trans youth as a valid and celebrated identity. This may be a long process. Support of the family, but also interacting with other families experiencing similar situations, may be a powerful way forward toward acceptance (Pullen Sansfaçon et al. 2015).

Underpinned by a commitment to uphold professional values, social workers also have the responsibility to challenge discrimination and promote diversity (IFSW 2012). In this sense, social workers' roles may be broader, and in cooperation with service users, and may involve challenging the environment that creates hardship and adversity that arise from strict social gender norms or other beliefs that lead to stigmatisation and oppression of trans youth. Indeed, some young people will have to navigate social environments that do not even recognise them legally, such as countries that do not allow young people to make their gender markers coherent with their gender identity. In such cases, young people will have to spend their childhood and teenage years with gender identity papers that are incoherent with who they are. This may affect the capacity for the young person to truly engage in civil society and lead to further social exclusion and discrimination. It then becomes difficult for them to live their lives according to their true gender identity since every time they are required to show some personal identification document, they are forced to do some coming out. This may lead to overt and covert discrimination, leading the young person to struggle, for example, in finding employment because of society's lack of acceptance of transgender identities; it may also lead young people to face transphobic violence, forcing them to be exposed as transgender people in the public sphere. There are countless examples of discrimination related to gender identity discrimination: at school, in the community, the passport a person travels with. Their experiences are constant reminders of discrimination and oppression.

When social workers get involved, they should take care to integrate all of these dimensions and attempt to support young people and families, but also challenge those structural and systemic barriers that contribute to their experience of adversity. This may be done by advocating for the young person at school so that their gender identity is honoured, or by having access to safe washrooms and changing rooms. It may involve social workers educating a youth club to help the neighbourhood environment be inclusive, or starting a support group for parents of gender non-conforming and transgender children so that they can better support each other, and challenge, by relying on their numbers, the oppressive structures that surround their children and their families. It may also mean social workers accompanying the child and their families in filing human-rights complaints so that discriminatory structures become inclusive of all young people (for an in-depth discussion of strategies to challenge discrimination and oppression, see Mullally 2010).

Conclusion

Social workers can play an important role in improving the well-being of transgender children and youth as well as their families. As the International Federation of Social Workers (2014) explains, social work "promotes social change and development, social cohesion, and the empowerment and liberation of people ... and engages people and structures to address life challenges and enhance well-being". Gender non-conforming children and trans youth are without a doubt a vulnerable group that can benefit from social work involvement. In this chapter, we have expressed and illustrated some of the main issues faced by trans children and youth, as well as by their families, and explored how that involvement can alleviate some of the difficulties. At the micro level, they can begin by supporting trans youth and their families in affirming their true gender identity, putting into place support services or referring the youth and families to them and supporting parents in the process of acceptance. We have also discussed how social workers can play a role in curbing stigmatisation and experiences of oppression faced by young people and their families. They can advocate on their behalf. By helping families get better support in the community, social workers can contribute to the well-being of young people affirming their identities, as well as work with families to facilitate parental acceptance, and more broadly, to contribute to social acceptance of trans youth and gender-diverse children.

Applying research findings to professional practice

- Regularly undertake introspection and critical analysis of your own values and social position as well as its impact on understanding gender and building relationship with transgender youth and their families.

- Drawing from social work values, critically analyse literature and evidence based publications on gender and trans-identities and the suggested way forward for intervention.
- Support and truly embrace young peoples' affirmed gender by respecting their self-determination and believing in who they are. The only person who can assert his or her identity is the person him/herself.
- Understand that most difficulties faced by trans youth and their families are structural and, therefore, requires changes at social and systemic levels; at the same time, understand that the person may also experience gender dysphoria and may also require intervention at an individual level.
- Be ready to advocate with, or on behalf of, trans youth and their families and challenge oppression. This can take the form of challenging/developing structures or policies both at micro and macro levels.
- Remember that trans youth lives are complex, that experiences and trajectories are diverse and that interventions cannot follow a one-model-fits-all mold. Analysis needs to take into account the various social locations (class, gender, age, "race", disability, etc.) of the young person and intervention being tailored-made accordingly, always prioritising the wishes and need of each individual young person.

References

Ajeto, D.M. (2009) *A Soul Has No Gender: Love and Acceptance through the Eyes of a Mother of Sexual and Gender Minority Children*. Rotterdam, Sense Publishers.
American Psychiatric Association (APA). (2013) *Gender Dysphoria*. (online) www.dsm5.org/documents/gender%20dysphoria%20fact%20sheet.pdf.
Bauer, G.R., et al. (2013) Suicidality among Trans People in Ontario: Implications for Social Work and Social Justice, *Service Social* 59 (1), 35–62.
Bauermeister, J.A., Johns, M.M., Sandfort, T.G.M., Eisenberg, A., Grossman, A.H., D'Augelliet, A.R. (2010) Relationship Trajectories and Psychological Well-Being among Sexual Minority Youth, *Journal of Youth and Adolescence* 39 (10), 1148–63.
Beemyn, B.G., Rankin, S. (2011) *The Lives of Transgender People*. New York, Columbia University Press.
Bith-Melander, P., Sheoran, B., Sheth, L, Bermudez., C., Drone, J., Wood, W., Schroeder, K. (2010) Understanding Sociocultural and Psychological Factors Affecting Transgender People of Color in San Francisco, *Journal of the Association of Nurses in AIDS Care*, Special Issue: Transgender Health and HIV Care Part II, 21 (3), 207–20.
Blumenfeld, W.J., Cooper, R.M. (2010) LGBT and Allied Youth Responses to Cyberbullying: Policy Implications, *The International Journal of Critical Pedagogy* 3 (1) 114–33.
Brennan, J., Kuhns, L.M., Johnson, A.K., Belzer, M., Wilson, E.C., Garofaloet, R. (2012) Syndemic Theory and HIV-Related Risk among Young Transgender Women: The Role of Multiple, Co-Occurring Health Problems and Social Marginalization, *American Journal of Public Health* 102 (9), 1751–57.

Brill, S., Pepper, R., (2013) *The Transgender Child: A Handbook for Families and Professionals*. California: Cleiss Press.

Bryant, K. (2006) Making Gender Identity Disorder of Childhood: Historical Lessons for Contemporary Debates, *Sexuality Research & Social Policy* 3 (3), 23–39.

Burgess, C. (2000) Internal and External Stress Factors Associated with the Identity Development of Transgendered Youth, *Journal of Gay & Lesbian Social Services* 10 (3–4), 35–47.

Canadian Association of Social workers. (2015) *Joint Statement on the Affirmation of Gender Diverse Children and Youth*. www.casw-acts.ca/en/joint-statement-affirmation-gender-diverse-children-and-youth.

Canadian Press. (2016) *Transgender Child's Puberty-Blocking Drug Triggers B.C. Supreme Court fight*. 28th April 2016, www.cbc.ca/news/canada/british-columbia/transgender-puberty-treatment-court-1.3556898.

Clark, T.C., Lucassen, M.F., Bullen, P., Denny, S.J., Fleming, T.M., Robinson, E.M., Rossen, F.V. (2014) The Health and Well-Being of Transgender Hight School Students: Results from the New Zealand Adolescent Health Survey, *Journal of Adolescent Health* 55 (1), 93–99.

Cochran, B.N., Stewart, A.J., Ginzler, J.A., Cauce, A.M. (2002) Challenges Faced by Homeless Sexual Minorities: Comparison of Gay, Lesbian, Bisexual, and Transgender Homeless Adolescents with Their Heterosexual Counterparts, *American Journal of Public Health* 92 (5), 773–77.

Cohen-Kettenis, P.T., Schagen, S.E., Steensma, T.D., de Vries, A.L.C., Delemarre-van de Waaland, H F. (2011) Puberty Suppression in a Gender-Dysphoric Adolescent: A 22-Year Follow-Up, *Archives of Sexual Behavior* 40 (4), 843–47.

Cook-Daniels, L. (2011) Social change and justice for all: The role of SOFFAs in the trans community (CLAGS). *Trans Politics, Social Change, and Justice*, Center for Lesbian and Gay Studies, New York, City University of New York.

Crossley, S. (2015) Come out Come out Wherever You Are: A Content Analysis of Homeless Transgender Youth in Social Service Literature, *PSU McNair Scholars Online Journal* 9 (1), 1–14.

DeHaan, S., Kuper, L.E., Magee, J.C., Bigelow, L., Mustanski, B.S., (2013) The Interplay between Online and Offline Explorations of Identity, Relationships, and Sex: A Mixed-Methods Study with LGBT Youth, *The Journal of Sex Research* 50 (5), 421–34.

De Vries, A., Cohen-Kettenis, P. (2012) Clinical Management of Gender Dysphoria in Children and Adolescent. The Dutch Approach, *Journal of Homosexuality* 59(3), 301–20.

DiNovo, C. (2015) *Affirming Sexual Orientation and Gender Identity Act, Chapter 18 of the Statutes of Ontario*, 2015. www.ontla.on.ca/web/committee-proceedings/committee_transcripts_details.do?locale=en&BillID=3197&detailPage=/committee-proceedings/transcripts/files_html/03-JUN-2015_JP006.htm&ParlCommID=9000&Business=&Date=2015-06-03&DocumentID=29207 [accessed 28 September 2015].

DiFulvio, G.T. (2011) Sexual Minority Youth, Social Connection and Resilience: From Personal Struggle to Collective Identity, *Social Science & Medicine* 72 (10), 1611–17.

Drescher, J., Byne, W. (2012) The Treatment of Gender Dysphoric / Gender Variant Children and Adolescent, *Journal of Homosexuality* 59 (3), 295–300.

Durso, L.E., Gates, G.J. (2012) *Serving Our Youth: Findings from a National Survey of Services Providers Working with Lesbian, Gay, Bisexual and Transgender Youth Who Are Homeless or At Risk of Becoming Homeless.* Los Angeles, CA, The Williams Institute, The True Colors Fund, and The Palette.

Ehrensaft, D. (2011) *Gender Born, Gender Made: Raising Health Gender Non-Conforming Children.* New York, The Experiment, LLC.

Ehrensaft, D. (2014a) From Gender Identity Disorder to Gender Identity Creativity: The Liberation of Gender Non-Conforming Children and Youth, in *Supporting Transgender and Gender Creative Youth: Schools, Families, and Communities in Action*, eds. Elizabeth J. Meyer and Annie Pullen Sansfaçon, 1st edition. New York, Peter Lang Publishing, pp. 13–25.

Ehrensaft, D. (2014b) Found in Transition: Our Littlest Transgender People, *Contemporary Psychoanalysis* 50 (4), 571–92.

Garnette, L., et al. (2011) Lesbian, Gay, Bisexual, and Transgender (LGBT) Youth and the Juvenile Justice System, in *Juvenile Justice: Advancing Research, Policy, and Practice*, eds. Francine T. Sherman and Francine H. Jacobs. Hoboken, NJ, John Wiley & Sons, Inc, pp. 156–73.

Glenn, W. D. (2000). Reflections of an Emerging Male-to-Female Transgendered Consciousness. *Journal of Gay & Lesbian Social Services* 10 (3–4), 83–94.

Grossman, A.H., D'Augelli, A.R. (2006) Transgender Youth: Invisible and Vulnerable, *Journal of Homosexuality* 51 (1), 111–28.

Grossman, A.H., D'Augelli, A.R., Frank, J.A. (2011) Aspects of Psychological Resilience among Transgender Youth, *Journal of LGBT Youth* 8 (2), 103–15.

Hegarty, P. (2009) Toward an LGBT-Informed Paradigm for Children Who Break Gender Norms: Comment on Drummond et al. (2008) and Rieger et al. (2008), *Developmental Psychology* 45 (4), 895–900.

Hellen, M. (2009). Transgender Children in Schools. *Liminalis: Journal for Sex/Gender Emancipation and Resistance* 9 (3), 81–99.

International Federation of Social Workers (2012) Statement of Ethical Principles. http://ifsw.org/policies/statement-of-ethical-principles/ [last accessed 19 January 2018]

Liu, R.T., Mustanski, B. (2012) Suicidal Ideation and Self-Harm in Lesbian, Gay, Bisexual, and Transgender Youth, *American Journal of Preventive Medicine* 42 (3), 221–28.

Magee, J.C., Bigelow, L., DeHaan, S., Mustanski, B.S. (2012) Sexual Health Information Seeking Online: A Mixed-Methods Study among Lesbian, Gay, Bisexual, and Transgender Young People, *Health Education & Behavior* 39 (3), 276–89.

Mallon, G.P. (2009) Summary of the Recommendations for clinical treatment of transgender and Gender Variant Youth, in *Social Work Practice with Transgender and Gender Variant Youth*, ed. G.P. Mallon. New York, Routledge.

Meadow, T. (2011) 'Deep down Where the Music Plays': How Parents Account for Childhood Gender Variance, *Sexualities* 14 (6), 725–47.

Menvielle, E. (2012) A Comprehensive Program for Children with Gender Variant Behaviors and Gender Identity Disorders, *Journal of Homosexuality* 59 (3), 357–68.

Mustanski, B., Liu, R.T. (2012) A Longitudinal Study of Predictors of Suicide Attempts among Lesbian, Gay, Bisexual, and Transgender Youth, *Archives of Sexual Behavior* 42 (3), 437–48.

Newcomb, M.E., Heinz, A.J., Mustanski, B. (2012) Examining Risk and Protective Factors for Alcohol Use in Lesbian, Gay, Bisexual, and Transgender Youth: A Longitudinal Multilevel Analysis, *Journal of Studies on Alcohol and Drugs* 73 (5), 783–93.

Nuttbrock, L., et al. (2010) Psychiatric Impact of Gender-Related Abuse across the Life Course of Male-to-Female Transgender Persons, *The Journal of Sex Research* 47 (1), 12–23.

Nuttbrock, L., et al. (2012) Gender Abuse, Depressive Symptoms, and HIV and Other Sexually Transmitted Infections among Male-to-Female Transgender Persons: A Three-Year Prospective Study, *American Journal of Public Health* 103 (2), 300–307.

Olson, J., Forbes, C., Belzer, M. (2011) Management of the Transgender Adolescent, *Archives of Pediatrics & Adolescent Medicine* 165 (2), 171–76.

Olson, K.R., Durwood, L., DeMeules, M., Mclaughlin, K.A. (2016) Mental Health of Transgender Children Who Are Supported in Their Identities, *Pediatrics* 137 (3), 2015–3223.

Olson, K.R., Key, A.C., Eaton, N.R. (2015) Gender Cognition in Transgender Children, *Psychological Sciences* 26 (4), 467–74.

Poirier, J.M., Fisher, S.K., Hunt, R.A., Bearse, M. (2014). *A Guide for Understanding, Supporting, and Affirming LGBTQI2-S Children, Youth, and Families.* Washington, DC, American Institutes for Research.

Price Minter, S. (2012) Supporting Transgender Children: New Legal, Social, and Medical Approaches, *Journal of Homosexuality* 59 (3), 422–33.

Pullen Sansfaçon, A. (2015) Parentalité et Jeunes Transgenres: Un Survol Des Enjeux Vécus et Des Interventions À Privilégier Pour Le Développement de Pratiques Transaffirmatives, *Santé Mentale Au Québec* 40 (3), 93–107.

Pullen Sansfaçon, A., Meyer, E.J., Manning K., Robichaud, M.J. (2014) Looking Back, Looking Forward, in *Supporting Transgender and Gender Creative Youth: Schools, Families, and Communities in Action*, eds. Elizabeth J. Meyer and Annie Pullen Sansfaçon, 1st edition. New York, Peter Lang Publishing, pp. 207–16.

Pullen Sansfaçon, A., Robichaud, M.J., Dumais-Michaud, A.A. (2015) The Experience of Parents Who Support Their Children's Gender Variance, *Journal of LGBT Youth* 12 (1), 39–63.

Pyne (2014) in *Supporting Transgender and Gender Creative Youth: Schools, Families, and Communities in Action*, ed. Elizabeth J. Meyer and Annie Pullen Sansfaçon, 1st edition. New York, Peter Lang Publishing Inc.

Riggs, D., Due, C. (2015) Support Experiences and Attitudes of Australian Parents of Gender Variant Children, *Journal of Child Families Studies* 24 (7), 1999–2007.

Riley, E.A., Sitharthan, G., Clemson, L., Diamond, M. (2011). The Needs of Gender Variant and their Parents: A Parent Survey, *International Journal of Sexual Health* 23 (2), 181–95.

Riley, E.A., Sitharthan, G., Clemson, L., Diamond, M. (2013). Surviving a Gender Variant Childhood: The Views of Transgender Adults on the Needs of Gender Variant Children and their Parents, *Journal of Sex & Marital Therapy* 39 (3), 241–62.

Roberts, A.E., et al. (2012) Childhood Gender Nonconformity: A Risk Indicator for Childhood Abuse and Posttraumatic Stress in Youth, *Pediatrics* 129 (3), 410–17.

Saketopoulou, A. (2011) Minding the Gap: Intersections between Gender, Race, and Class in Work with Gender Variant Children, *Psychoanalytic Dialogues* 21 (2), 192–209.

Sifra Quintana, N., Rosenthal, J., Krehely, J (2010) *On the Streets: The Federal Response to Gay and Transgender Homeless Youth*. Washington, DC, Center for American Progress.

Singh, A.A. (2012) Transgender Youth of Color and Resilience: Negotiating Oppression and Finding Support, *Sex Roles* 68 (11–12), 690–702.

Singh, A.A., Meng, S.E., Hansen, A.W. (2014) 'I Am My Own Gender': Resilience Strategies of Trans Youth, *Journal of Counseling & Development* 92 (2), 208–18.

Stieglitz, K.A. (2010) Development, Risk, and Resilience of Transgender Youth, *Journal of the Association of Nurses in AIDS Care*, Special Issue: Transgender Health and HIV Care Part II, 21 (3), 192–206.

Stroumsa, D. (2014) The State of Transgender Health Care: Policy, Law, and Medical Frameworks, *American Journal of Public Health* 104 (3), 31–38.

Testa, H., Hendrick, M.L. (2015) Suicide Risk among Transgender and Gender Non-conforming Youth, pp 121–131 in *Youth Suicide and Bullying*, eds. Peter Goldblum, Dorothy L. Espelage, Joyce Chui, and Bruce Bongar. New York, Oxford University Press, pp. 121–31.

Travers, R., Bauer, G., Pyne, J., Bradley, K. (2012) *Impact of Strong Parental Support for Trans Youth*. Toronto, ON, TRANS Pulse Report.

Torres Bernal, A., Coolhart, D. (2012) Treatment and Ethical Considerations with Transgender Children and Youth in Family Therapy, *Journal of Family Psychotherapy* 23 (4), 287–303.

Walls, N.E., Bell, S. (2011) Correlates of Engaging in Survival Sex among Homeless Youth and Young Adults, *Journal of Sex Research* 48 (5), 423–36.

Wallace, R., Russell, H. (2013) Attachment and Shame in Gender-Nonconforming Children and Their Families: Toward a Theoretical Framework for Evaluating Clinical Interventions, *International Journal of Transgenderism* 14 (3), 113–26.

Wilson, E.C., Iverson, E., Garofalo, R., Belzer, M. (2012) Parental Support and Condom Use among Transgender Female Youth, *Journal of the Association of Nurses in AIDS Care* 23 (4), 306–17.

World Professional Association of Transgender Care (WPATH). (2011) Standards of care for the Health of Transsexual, Transgender, and Gender Nonconforming People, Version 7.

Wren, B. (2002). 'I Can Accept My Child Is Transsexual but If I Ever See Him in a Dress I'll Hit Him': Dilemmas in Parenting a Transgendered Adolescent, *Clinical Child Psychology and Psychiatry* 7 (3), 377–97.

Wyss, S.E. (2004) 'This Was My Hell': The Violence Experienced by Gender Non-Conforming Youth in US High Schools, *International Journal of Qualitative Studies in Education* 17 (5), 709–30.

Zucker, K.J., Wood, H., Singh, D., Bradley, S. (2012) A Developmental, Biopsychosocial Model for the Treatment of Children with Gender Identity Disorder, *Journal of Homosexuality* 59 (3), 369–97.

3 Combatting homophobic and transphobic bullying in schools through family engagement

Trish Hafford-Letchfield, Christine Cocker, Peter Ryan, Mary Martin, Rosalind Scott and Sarah Carr

Introduction

This chapter draws on findings from a European project, 'Rights through alliances: Innovating and networking both within homes and schools' (RAINBOW-HAS), conducted during 2013–2015. RAINBOW-HAS involved collaboration between six European Union countries to analyse and improve the rights of children, young people and their families experiencing bullying in relation to sexual and gender identities in educational settings (Arateko, 2015). We share some of the key findings emerging from a review of the education policy literature on homophobic and transphobic bullying in the UK, and then use this to foreground a practice example led by the English project team which developed and piloted a family and student led intervention within two secondary schools aimed at preventing homophobic and transphobic bullying. We reflect on the potential of such an intervention as a model for community engagement with secondary schools and lesbian, gay, bisexual and transgender (LGBT) young people and their families. Finally, we discuss the implications for social work where there is tendency for silence on LGBT issues more broadly and conclude with some suggestions for how social workers can be more active in their contribution to young people's well-being in education through LGBT rights-based advocacy.

The European context for LGBT rights

Discrimination on the grounds of sexual orientation is prohibited both by article 13 of the Treaty of the European Union (2012) and European Charter of Fundamental Rights (2000) alongside equality legislation and national constitutions established by Europe's individual member states. Two reports published by the Council of Europe (ILGA-Europe, 2015) and internationally (Amnesty International, 2014), have sought to raise the profile of people from the LGBT community. These fundamental activities combined with successful social movements on LGBT rights signal a stronger LGBT agenda in Europe. However, there is still a significant gap between the legislation and institutions in the EU member states and the actual conditions and circumstances of LGBT individuals and their communities on the ground (ILGA-Europe, 2015) and there is a lack of robust, comparable data on the respect, protection and fulfilment of the fundamental rights of LGBT people in relation to discrimination and hate crimes.

RAINBOW-HAS (Rights through alliances: Innovating and networking both within homes and schools) was co-funded by the Fundamental Rights and Citizenship Programme of the EU. Collaboration between participating institutions specifically: Ararteko (ES) (Project co-ordinator): Akademia Pedagogiki Specjalnej Marii Grzegorzewskiej (PL), Associació de Famílies Lesbianes i Gais de Catalunya (ES), Comune di Milano (IT), ECIP Foundation (BG), Farapi (ES), Jekino Educatie vzw (BE), Middlesex University Higher Education Corporation (UK), Synergia (IT) (Project partners): COC Amsterdam (NL), Gemeente Amsterdam (NL), LSVD (DE), Centro di Iniziativa Gay Onlus (IT), University of East Anglia (UK) (Project associate). These research centres were located across six European Union countries, (Bulgaria, Belgium, Italy, Poland, Spain and the UK) and investigated homophobic bullying across schools in five of these countries (not Belgium).

Research indicates that homophobic, transphobic and heteronormative bullying within education has severe consequences for children and young people's safety and well-being (Tippett et al., 2010; Smith et al., 2014). Education and schools, in particular, are known to make a difference (Birkett et al., 2009). There is, however, a relative silence from the profession on this issue (Mishna et al., 2009; Cocker and Hafford-Letchfield, 2010), despite the potential role it plays in the provision of proper, safe and supportive spaces for children, young people and their families and carers (Guasp, 2010; Hafford-Letchfield et al., 2016). Freedom from discrimination and harm is essential to be able to learn, develop and flourish (Rivers, 2001; Adams et al., 2004; DePalma and Atkinson, 2009; Monk, 2009). Schools are also potentially influential institutions in combating humiliating stereotypes or the perpetuation of prejudice fostering social exclusion, discrimination or the denial of human dignity (Adams et al., 2014). Whilst anti-bullying intervention programmes have been implemented in the last three decades on a large scale in Europe (Farrington and Ttofi, 2010) and internationally (UNESCO, 2012), little cross-national learning has occurred. Non-targeted anti-bullying interventions in schools for LGBT children and youth may also be hampered by deficits in a nation's broader socio-legal context for homophobia, heterosexism and heteronormativity (Walton, 2006) and impacts on all children, not just those experiencing it. There is more to learn from research into the multifaceted nature of bullying in the education environment, in terms of the roles played by teachers, parents and carers, social workers and other children and how different types of bullying are conceptualised and addressed.

RAINBOW-HAS looked at how its participating countries responded to these diverse issues and provided opportunities for cross-fertilisation of ideas within a context where there are different legislation and policies, institutions, cultures as well as socio-economic and political differences.

Whilst each participating country had a different starting point, there were many commonalities. Good practice was not just associated with advanced development, but in finding ways to tackle issues within countries that are geographically and culturally varied. Alongside building a transnational community, RAINBOW-HAS brought important concepts from Europe into the individual domestic contexts through its direct engagement with young people and their families. Given that homophobic and transphobic bullying has become a legitimate object of social concern within civil society, RAINBOW-HAS asked critical questions about bullying from young people and their carers' own perspectives. These are important for social workers not generally situated in educational environments, but working with those affected. By placing bullying that takes place at school within a broader political and cultural context, these perspectives help to conceptualise bullying within education primarily as a discourse as opposed to simply harm (see Monk, 2009).

There were a number of outcomes from the RAINBOW-HAS initiatives which have already been reported elsewhere (see Ararteko, 2015; Hafford-Letchfield et al., 2016; Cocker et al., 2018). These involved a synthesis of themes and findings which, whilst providing only a snapshot of contemporary practice across the European context, generated some interesting cross comparative and discursive analysis of the experiences of LGBT parents, their relationships with school communities and a wide range of strategies in each participating country to address homophobic and transphobic bullying. Given the amount of data generated and the complexity of narratives present within and between each country's samples, developing a targeted and comprehensive approach to homophobic and transphobic bullying presented complex challenges. The remainder of this chapter looks at the context for the English in-country research. We summarise some of the key findings from the biblio-sitography of the UK context and refer to some of the specific themes from the English data as a result of RAINBOW-HAS. Finally, we provide a short case study on our experience of developing and implementing a family and student led intervention within two secondary schools in an effort to demonstrate some leadership in acknowledging, recognising and responding to this specific form of bullying.

Themes from the UK biblio-sitography

Homophobic bullying within the UK has only been taken relatively seriously in the last decade within the parameters of policies and actions of bullying in schools generally. It is important to recap some of the underlying contributing factors to why this is the case. Section 28 of the Local Government Act 1988, which was finally repealed in 2003 in England and Wales, appeared to confuse many schools about how to address LGBT issues within their schools, and this served to reinforce the silence surrounding the subject. Section 28 demanded that a Local Authority 'must not "promote homosexuality" or "promote the teaching in any maintained school of the acceptability of homosexuality as a *pretend* family relationship'". Whilst a government circular from the Department of the Environment Circular (1988: 12/88) had made it clear that 'Section 28 does not affect the activities of school governors nor of teachers. It will not prevent the objective discussion of homosexuality in the classroom, nor the counselling of students, concerning their sexuality' (section 20), there had been general confusion and lack of clarity amongst schools about their responsibilities towards issues of homophobia and preventing any initiatives in gaining ground. In 1994, the report of an Anti-Bullying Project was funded by the UK Government Department for Education (DfE, 2000) resulting in the development of a guidance pack for schools called *Don't Suffer in Silence*, based on its findings. This was a significant publication for Government policy discourse which has since regarded bullying in schools as a key priority. It wasn't until the introduction of the Schools Standards and Framework Act (HMG, 1998) that a legal requirement for schools to have an Anti-Bullying Policy (as part of a Pupil Discipline Policy) was subsequently introduced in 1999. The Charter for Action (Department for Children, Education and Skills, 2004) following from the Education Act 2002 has since required schools and Local Authorities to actively safeguard and promote the welfare of children, and this includes responding to bullying. It is important to note however that homophobic or transphobic bullying was not specifically highlighted within these developments.

Two significant research briefs (DfES, 2003a, 2003b) on tackling bullying which engaged with the views of children and young people highlighted the damage that bullying can do to young people and their educational and social achievements, and it wasn't until 2005 when the Governments Behaviour Tsar (DfES, 2005) made a specific recommendation on tackling bullying motivated by prejudice including homophobia, racism and persecution in all its various manifestations. The Education and Inspections Act 2006 also gave head teachers the ability to respond to incidents that take place outside of school hours, for example, on public transport, or via mobile phones and the internet (cyberbullying). Further, governing bodies within schools are legally responsible for acts of discrimination, harassment and victimisation carried out by school staff, regardless of whether they knew about or approved of those acts.

In 2007, the UK Government held a national inquiry through its Select Committee into bullying (House of Commons, 2007), taking evidence from a range of individuals and organisations involved in the development or delivery of anti-bullying programmes. They included schools, campaigning organisations and support organisations, and the inquiry explored the barriers that prevent schools from tackling bullying effectively. This included areas such as prejudice-driven bullying, Special Educational Needs-related, homophobic, faith-based and cyberbullying. It also sought to address the lack of research on how bullying affects bullies, given suggestions that there may be significant problems for individuals and the community generally if bullying behaviour which occurs in childhood is not tackled and changed. A key definition was also put forward:

> Repetitive, wilful or persistent behaviour intended to cause harm, although one-off incidents can in some cases also be defined as bullying; Intentionally harmful behaviour, carried out by an individual or a group; and resulting in an imbalance of power leaving the person being bullied feeling defenceless. Bullying is emotionally or physically harmful behaviour and includes: name-calling; taunting; mocking; making offensive comments; kicking; hitting; pushing; taking belongings; inappropriate text messaging and emailing; sending offensive or degrading images by phone or via the internet; gossiping; excluding people from groups and spreading hurtful and untruthful rumours.
>
> (DfES, 2007)

> Teachers unions and professional organisations such as the National Association of Students and National Union of Teachers have been active in providing revised strategies and guidance on dealing with LGBT bullying.
>
> (NUT, 2017)

Prejudice-driven bullying

A distinctive feature of prejudice-driven bullying is that a person is attacked not only as an individual, but also as the representative of a family, community or group resulting in other members of the same group, family or community being or feeling threatened and/or intimidated. This has wider social implications, extending beyond the school setting and schools. This was an important tenet within the RAINBOW-HAS research where lesbian and gay parents were interviewed about the experiences of their children and themselves in relation to school integration as a result of having different families. This is illustrated in the quote from one of the lesbian parents interviewed below (Cocker et al., 2018):

> The last parents evening... we met the physics teacher. We sat down and we said we're X's mothers. And he was like [makes a face] 'I don't understand'. I said 'what don't you understand?' We were sitting down by this stage. He said, 'Why X has got two mothers?'... I then replied, 'We're in a civil partnership and X's our daughter'. 'Physics is very difficult anyway' he said. The next day I called the head of year who is fabulous and gay himself and he said 'that is my jaw hitting the desk... what can I say, he's a physics teacher'. I said, 'I'm not making a complaint but perhaps someone needs to have a word with him to bring him up to date'. He said 'absolutely'.
>
> (Family 5)

Here we can see how parents are made to do the work on challenging homophobia in schools and how action and inaction has significance in limiting or bypassing the negative consequences of homophobic attitudes on wider society. This example compliments other research demonstrating that teachers are less certain in dealing with name-calling and other verbal abuse about sexuality than any other matter (Ofsted, 2002). Students also find this area difficult where it is common for their peers to make personal comments about others' sexuality, such as using the expression 'you're gay', using a condemnatory, homophobic tone. These statements may be dismissed as being simply silly, but for those trying to make sense of their own sexuality; this can contribute to a climate marked by crude stereotyping and hostility to difference. Current government guidance to schools however is that they should involve the entire school community in agreeing on a definition of bullying and it is recommended that additional guidance is given to schools on how to ensure difficult issues, such as the use of homophobic language and more subtle forms of bullying, are included in this process. Young people may see identity-related bullying as worse than general bullying because identity related bullying focused on things that could not be changed. Within the findings from RAINBOW-HAS, sexuality alongside race, culture and disability was one thing that respondents mentioned in relation to identity-related bullying (Hafford-Letchfield et al., 2016; Cocker et al., 2018) echoing the findings of the Select Committee (2007) that prejudice-driven bullying is different from other forms of bullying and requires targeted attention.

Stonewall (2017) whose national initiative and campaign on homophobic bullying in education (Schools Out) suggest that the degree of isolation is greater for the victims of homophobic bullying because they may have to 'come out' in order to report the bullying. While this may be part of the reason young people who experience homophobic bullying do not report it, there are challenges in being able to speak easily to a teacher about bullying as well as finding sympathetic peers. Friendship and social status have been another area where evidence suggests both a protective factor and a risk factor (British Psychological Society, 2014). Victims are often at greater 'social risk' as they lack supportive friends at schools and tend to be more rejected by their peers. The School Report 2017, a study of over 3,700 lesbian, gay, bi and trans (LGBT) pupils across Britain, demonstrates the continued impact of this work. Since the 2007 School Report, the number of lesbian, gay and bi pupils bullied because of their sexual orientation has fallen by almost a third. The number of schools who say this bullying is wrong has nearly trebled, and homophobic remarks are far less likely to be heard. Hunt and Jensen (2007) in a survey of 1,100 young people found that homophobic bullying was highest in religious schools. This is an area that Stonewall has also tried to address in working with faith communities and they cite a number of good practice examples in their guides written for an education audience (Stonewall, 2017). Ninety-eight per cent of young LGB persons hear phrases such as 'that's so gay' used in a pejorative way, and 97 per cent hear insulting remarks such as 'poof', 'dyke', and 'rug-muncher'. They also documented the following forms of harassment: Verbal abuse (92 per cent), physical abuse (41 per cent), cyberbullying (41 per cent), death threats (17 per cent) and sexual assault (12 per cent). However, the RAINBOW-HAS research found that it is difficult to determine the extent of bullying due to lack of record keeping and problems with establishing a consistent definition (Ararteko, 2015). The schools involved in interviews identified that attention was often given to the person bullied rather than the bully, and where pupils came out, they may sometimes be told by teachers to keep their head down and not draw attention to themselves. Little is known about the teachers and their own experiences of homophobic bullying. Lesbian and gay parents interviewed during the RAINBOW-HAS project reported being aware of teachers at their children's school who were members of the LGBT community but were not able to be 'out', which they found to be very contradictory when the parents were involved in raising the profile of homophobic bullying within their own schools (Hafford-Letchfield et al., 2016; Cocker et al., 2018).

> I spoke to the chair of governors, and I'm going to have a blitz on the new head so that teachers feel comfortable coming out. It's a relatively small number of people, and could be to do with the people they have got (the teachers who are gay), but there are things that could be done to get people in the school to make those connections.
>
> (Family 2)

Other themes from the research literature have highlighted the importance of challenging homophobic attitudes and the inclusion of homophobia within the school curriculum, which has also been picked up the statutory regulatory body, Ofsted. They drew on inspections and surveys with 140 primary, secondary and special schools, discussions with 650 young people, postal surveys of 1,000 primary, secondary and special schools in 20 local educational authorities, and meetings with education and health professionals (Ofsted, 2012). They identified that schools' different interpretations of their aims and values produced confusions regarding what was deemed acceptable and unacceptable. Ofsted commented that this could result in homophobic attitudes going unchallenged in too many schools and derogatory terms about homosexuality being part of everyday practice. Adams et al. (2004) also investigated how effectively issues of homophobic bullying and sexualities were addressed through secondary schools' formal policies and areas of the curriculum within 19 secondary schools. The outcomes of their small scale research indicated that whilst sexual orientation was mentioned in two-thirds of equal opportunities policies, it was not mentioned specifically in any anti-bullying policies. Staff highlighted the need for training in issues surrounding sexualities, homophobic bullying and clarification of Section 28 (as this was in place at the time of their study).

The data collected for RAINBOW-HAS in the English workstream included interviews and surveying best practice initiatives of schools who saw themselves as being active in promoting LGBT issues in their curriculum.

One example was a London based secondary school which has grappled with this issue successfully. They provided an illustration of how they developed content on gay historical figures who suffered persecution, such as Oscar Wilde (literary figure) and Andy Warhol (artist), which they suggested has succeeded in 'more or less eliminating homophobic bullying' in its classrooms and playgrounds over the last five years (Shepherd and Learner, 2010). The school has subsequently developed a training package for primary and secondary school teachers in how to 'educate and celebrate' being gay.

More recently McDermott (2010) attempted to systematically capture evidence on the disadvantages experienced by young people due to their sexual orientation such as homophobic bullying, mental health issues, rejection from family and friends and increased risk of homelessness. The extent and impact of this disadvantage has not been systematically examined or analysed to date and constitutes a major evidence gap. Equally, McDermott has asserted that a first step in understanding how to capture such inequality is to review the evidence and explore the issues involved in researching and monitoring sexual orientation in adolescence. For example, where young people are beginning to recognise and deal with emerging sexual feelings and attraction to others, some may be more certain whilst others remain unsure about their sexual orientation. McDermott suggests that where young people also begin to identify the actual/perceived sexual orientation of others, this can underpin homophobic bullying. Targeting health or education interventions for young people during these vulnerable periods could help to ensure the safety and well-being of all young people, whatever their sexual orientation.

In summary, the development of positive action towards incidences of homophobic and transphobic bullying has been slow to develop and more research is needed on how sexual and gender diversities may intersect with other dimensions of disadvantage, such as disabilities, ethnicity, social class and gender, within the school environment. This is especially important given the provision in the UK Equality Act (HMG, 2010) to protect people on the basis of combined protected characteristics. Further research needs to be more sophisticated and develop questions and methods capable of capturing this intersectionality. Since 2012 all schools in England and Wales were required to publish their equality objectives, explaining how they intend to meet these duties (DfE, 2013), including those published in the government's White Paper (2010) *The Importance of Teaching* (DfE, 2010), which highlighted their responsibility to prevent and respond to homophobic bullying.

Developing practice initiatives from RAINBOW-HAS: a case study

The above review of the literature, policy background and other evidence, including examples from RAINBOW-HAS, provides the background to the final section of this chapter, which briefly describes an intervention piloted by two schools in the RAINBOW-HAS UK partnership. Lesbian and gay parents who participated in the study described the notion of being both insiders and outsiders in school communities depending on whose voices were dominant or subverted in this environment. Their narratives also revealed blame and survival strategies in relation to bullying behaviour and experiences, and discourses relating to the 'problematisation vs ordinariness of LGBT families' in a heteronormative world (see Hafford-Letchfield et al., 2016; Cocker et al., 2018). Further, interviews conducted with head teachers and other education staff leading on bullying initiatives in English schools revealed that whilst some progress has been made, there was compelling evidence to show that homophobic and transphobic bullying in schools remains a highly problematic area in relation to other types of bullying. In order to make progress, there was a lot of discussion within the project team on the best way of targeting homophobic and transphobic bullying in schools in a way that would engage stakeholders who would feel less confident or with families who may not recognise or identify with the issues. Similarly, there was plenty of evidence of good practice, and these are summarised in Table 3.1 below.

Table 3.1 Examples of good practice from the school participants data

Examples of good practice from the interviews with primary and secondary schools (n = 4)
Teachers being aware and open to the potential of children in the school exploring their sexual identity and reinforcing different identities Comprehensive training programme to support staff knowledge and skills Working with Stonewall Champion programme and learning materials Use of inclusive day to day language by teachers – 'carers'and 'parents' instead of 'mum and dad' Children, staff and governors collaborating to form 'Equality' teams Forming an inclusive working party of students and teachers to write the school anti-bullying policy and promoting its progress through school assemblies Playground 'buddy' schemes Making short promotional films about bullying issues Designing and introducing a leaflet about homophobic language Ensuring age appropriate reading materials which promote different families (And Tango makes three) followed by activities to allow children to explore and engage with anti-bullying messages Hosting a week long 'Same Difference' diversity festival with homophobia as main theme Involving parents in celebrating LGBT history month Supporting LGBT teenagers to share their experiences with other students Hosting Pride Sports organisation to run workshops within the school Inviting famous gay actor to speak at the school Introducing students to Stonewall's Youth Volunteering programme Introducing a log for recording when and where the word gay was used in derogatory terms and monitoring and reviewing responses from teachers Developing an LGBT champions programme, appointing ambassadors and establishing an LGBT lunchtime club Developing a whole school ethos approach to diversity which recognises and connects different types of diversity and discrimination

Data from four schools participating in 'best practice' interviews and who also provided case studies of students subject to homophobic and transphobic bullying also identified a number of challenges for schools promoting LGBT issues, particularly for those serving ethnically and religiously diverse and socially deprived communities. Here is a quote from one of the schools based in a large urban area:

> We had attempted to bring sex education into the schools as many of the young girls were coming into school menstruating and did not know what was happening. We wanted to teach them hygiene and about the changes happening to their body. It turned into a serious situation. We held a meeting with parents – psychologists and the local police were invited to attend as well. As head teacher I was expected to lead at the meeting and had been prepped on what to say but when I entered the meeting the hostility from the parents was so great I forgot everything I was supposed to say. Different groups of parents clashed as a father who was quite fundamentalist in his approach was hyping up the situation and saying the school was teaching gay sex, and then the Afro-Caribbean community said they wanted the sex education with no adaptations. We now tackle same sex relationships in a subtle way so they would not know that this is being incorporated into the curriculum.
>
> (Head Teacher)

Another example of the challenges is illustrated here:

> It was the most scared I have been here, 15 parents caught me in the playground and pointed me out saying 'he is the one' and they shouted at me, asking "why are you teaching our children about gay sex", 8 men harangued me. One man said if you teach my children about gay sex you will burn in hell.
>
> (Teacher)

In one school, for example, when teachers informed parents that it would be doing some specific work for LGBT History Month, a minority group of parents voiced concern. Three parents came into school and spoke with the head teacher. However, when the school management team showed them the books and the lesson plans that were going to be used, these parents commented that teaching about accepting difference was something they themselves agreed with and practiced at home – and were happy for their children to take part. The festival programme helped the school to build on an existing commitment to lesbian and gay equality by identifying areas for improvement. As a result, the school now stocks a range of books with lesbian and gay themes in their library and LGBT

History Month celebrations are now curriculum-wide with all subject areas delivering lessons with an LGBT theme. The school also used 'different families, same love' LGBT inclusive promotion posters from Stonewall's national campaign which helped to reinforce the variety of family relationships and types of families that could be in the school community.

The learning from these examples above provided by schools championing LGBT issues enabled the RAINBOW-HAS team in England to host two regional seminars involving local organisations and schools to discuss the empirical findings from families, schools and the literature review. These workshop consultations helped to inform the design and content of a training intervention which two school partners agreed to pilot. There were clear recommendations that any interventions should (a) be addressed by the educational community as a whole; (b) be developed in partnership with families and young people so as to encourage them to develop their own knowledge and skills needed to combat bullying and (c) take place at a point of transition from primary to secondary education which was seen as an important time where children are developing their identities and for parents represents a sensitive period making them more amenable to engagement on bullying issues so as to support their child's transition. Second, many parents and carers who do not consider that their child will either be subject or involved in perpetrating homophobic and transphobic bullying may not be primarily interested in these issues. Having a programme that targets this issue may not gain as much support as a programme that integrates the issues. This 'preaching to the converted' can make it difficult to get commitment to the topic as the following quote from a teacher illustrates:

> By looking at sexuality as part of our wider focus on equality, it was very easy for our young people to see the parallels with other forms of discrimination: if they agreed that racism was wrong and comments about people with disabilities were unacceptable, why should it be OK to treat someone differently because of their sexuality?
>
> (Teacher)

The workshops

Three 90 minute workshops were designed to bring together the children entering their first year of secondary school, their parents and teachers from their secondary school. Teachers were expected to model leadership roles in developing a culture of acceptance in the school, and the workshop coordinator drew on staff with a particular commitment and role in addressing bullying in its various forms, and homophobic bullying in particular.

These workshops focused on children entering secondary school in their first year of secondary education. They supported the establishment and maintenance of a culture of acceptance and the celebration of diversity with respect to a range of differences in gender, race, sexual orientation and disability. This embedding of partnership within a programme that addressed bullying in all its forms was designed to highlight the relationships between a broad range of bullying behaviour and in particular, homophobic bullying.

Participants included: parents of children aged around 11–12 who were entering their first year of secondary school education; children themselves from this age band; representatives of school and school executive team; and representatives of local community, where appropriate. The programme took place as an after-school activity to maximise participation and comprised three workshops, once a month over a three-month period in total. The provision of a suitable public space within the school environment was crucial, so teachers and families could meet up in a friendly, helpful and casual environment, which lended itself to developing a sense of collaboration.

Two sites piloted the intervention. Secondary school A was a co-educational academy school for students aged 11–18 years in the south-east region with approximately 1,370 students. It is a member of an Academy Trust and was originally founded in 1960. There were 36 participants in the training programme: 4 parents, 28 students/siblings and 4 teaching staff. Secondary school B was a co-educational academy for students aged 11–18 years in a rural area and had around 1,380 students. It is also an academy school. There were 25 participants in the training programme: 5 parents, 15 students/siblings and 5 teaching staff. The Head of Anti-Bullying and the Executive Principal also attended for some of the sessions.

The workshop programme and session structure

Table 3.2 provides an outline of the programme developed and used to guide the structure, content and process across the workshops, although these were adapted by the teams to their local circumstances.

In order to ensure that the student and their well-being was central to the workshops, the students were asked to construct a figure to represent someone who was coming to the school for the first time from primary school. The figure prompted students to reflect on and discuss the individual's experiences and feelings. Participants were then asked for their perspectives on different kinds of bullying, what causes bullying and how it happens. They were also asked what they thought could be done about it. Discussion and reflection exercises were facilitated by the

Table 3.2 Structure of the workshop programme

Task	Goal	Timing/duration
1 Brief period of social interaction as families/ school staff arrive and settle down	To orientate families, the school and any community stakeholders present to the main issues and themes being addressed in this dialogue between schools and families	5 minutes
2 Establishing and maintaining ground-rules including warm up exercises	To emphasise and reinforce the importance of a clear, safe, predictable emotional space for the group	5 minutes (longer in first session)
3 Workshop Exercises		
a) Construct (using a pipe cleaner) a stick figure of a student in the school and discuss the figure	To assist participants in the workshop to identify with the experience of being a student in the school	15 minutes
b) How does bullying happen?	To help workshop participants identify the causes of bullying in particular contexts	15 minutes
c) What kinds of bullying are there?	To locate homophobic bullying in the context of all kinds of bullying	15 minutes
d) What causes bullying?	To help participants understand what contributes towards causing bullying	15 minutes
4 Family & school sharing & feedback	To give each family, and school the opportunity to discuss issues raised in stage three	20 minutes
5 Action Planning	Participants decide: 1 What 2 When 3 Where 4 With whom 5 By when 6 Outcomes	20 minutes
6 Group closure through informal social interaction	A brief final period of social interaction, to emphasise the positives of what the session has covered, ending with refreshments if possible	10 minutes
7 Total time		120 minutes

trainers, and students in small groups recorded their thoughts on large sheets of paper (Figure 3.1).

Participants were then asked for their perspectives on different kinds of bullying, what causes bullying and how it happens. They were also asked

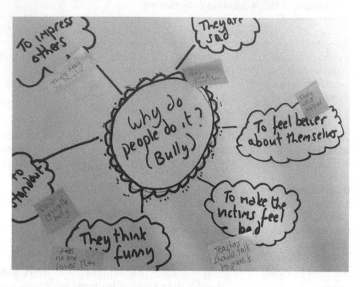

Figure 3.1 Snapshot of work generated by the teams.

what they thought could be done about it. Discussion and reflection exercises were facilitated by the trainers and students in small groups recorded their thoughts on large sheets of paper.

What kinds of bullying are there?

Across the two pilot sites the students identified four main types of bullying that young people encounter. These were verbal, physical and mental bullying, along with the increasingly prevalent 'cyberbullying' which occurs online and through social media such as Twitter or Facebook. Specific types of physical bullying mentioned were assault, spitting, pulling hair, 'hitting you, punching you or kicking you', vandalism or theft of the person's property and use of weapons (including dogs). Verbal bullying was experienced as teasing, banter, intimidation, impersonating or mocking the individual ('taking the mick'), threats, name-calling, swearing, 'laughing or jeering at you'. The types of 'mental' (psychological) bullying mentioned ranged from having 'fake friends', discrimination, 'ganging up on people', blackmail, isolation and peer pressure. Emotional bullying also focused on a person's appearance or through 'fake friends' and mistrust, 'being abandoned by friends and left alone'. Financial bullying was described as demanding money with threats. One particular form of cyberbullying was described as 'photo bullying' and circulating 'mug shots' through social media. Participants also focused on types of bullying based on the individual's characteristics and they were strongly aware of the effects of diversity and difference in bullying. The young people highlighted bullying associated with 'discrimination', racism, sexism and homophobia.

What causes bullying?

When asked to distinguish the causes of bullying, the students discussed both the characteristics of the bullied and the possible motivations of the bully. Again, diversity and difference in the bullied were strongly highlighted with students recording gender, race, age, sexuality, religion, disability or illness, appearance, personality, size and weight, skin colour, hair colour, accent, money and possessions, clothes, popularity, friendship groups, intelligence, facial features, background or nationality, interests and hobbies. One group simply summed the issue up by saying 'difference' while another identified being alone as a risk for being bullied. When considering the motivations of the bully, the students recorded a variety of possible reasons. Jealousy was the most consistently cited reason, followed by 'ignorance' and 'peer pressure'. Pleasure, superiority, boredom, fun, revenge, anger, hate, 'craving power', reputation, 'trying to impress others' and materialism were also given as reasons why bullies bully others. Being mistreated by family or friends or being bullied themselves was thought by some students to be a cause of bullying behaviour, with some also citing low self-esteem. One discussion group suggested the role of the media and television for influencing bullying was considerable. Most of the students also discussed the influence of psychological and situational factors on the bully's behaviour, with low self-esteem or self-image, stress and problems at home or in their background being cited in several discussions. Many emphasised the possibility that the bully could be themselves a victim of bullying or abuse, perhaps at home.

How does bullying happen?

Across both groups, some of the students in the discussion groups thought that 'gang mentality' enabled bullying to happen, while others thought that the bullying dynamic was about 'homing in on a weakness'. When considering the site of bullying, many of the students thought it could happen both in school and out of school, with some saying 'anywhere', particularly in the case of cyberbullying. Several students reflected on the serious mental health impacts of bullying, with one discussion group recording that it 'can lead to suicide or self-harm in the bullied'. The student discussion groups addressed the question of how bullying starts and suggested that 'rumour' and 'betrayal' are very common reasons. More specifically they said bullying can 'escalate from a joke or rumour' or 'making comments in school'. The joke or rumour can then be spread more rapidly through 'social media messaging' and end up 'getting taken too far'.

What helps prevent and tackle bullying in school?

Student participants identified a range of strategies and interventions to help prevent and tackle bullying. Some were concerned with the actions an individual might take if they are being bullied while some focused on how peers and friends should respond. The students wanted to encourage the bullied individual to disclose and report what was happening to them to family, friends and teachers (or 'head of college'). They advised that the individual should report bullying to the school ('school office') or the police, if necessary. Speaking to a trusted and understanding person was seen as an important first step, particularly to stop the isolation (some also recommended finding friends as a protective factor). Another commonly suggested tactic was to ignore the bullies (because getting upset would give them satisfaction) or to stand up to them. 'Being careful of social media' was also recommended. Peers and friends could be supportive through helping the bullied individual to tell someone and to support them. It was suggested that peers and friends could help with 'zero tolerance' of bullying and help prevent escalation by 'keeping an eye out'. One idea was to create 'mood' or 'thought' boxes to record and understand their emotional and psychological responses to instances of bullying.

The workshop participants were then asked about what students should expect from the school and they identified a range of strategies and approaches that could prevent and tackle bullying. There was a strong consensus that parents and schools should work together in partnership to tackle individual cases of bullying and to develop action plans and strategies. A culture of listening and communication between students, parents and the school, where all were taken seriously and treated with respect, was recognised as important. It was felt that students' voices need to be heard by parents and the school. Most were of the opinion that the school should be a safe environment for all students, where they are happy to be educated, 'socialise in a friendly way' and make friends. A safe school environment was thought to be enabled by 'all staff being against bullying'. Feeling safe also meant knowing which members of staff they could talk to with the certainty that they would be listened to and having reliable staff 'who can be trusted to act quickly on bullying'.

Operational and procedural aspects were identified as being important for addressing and preventing bullying. Having a 'good disciplinary system' or bullying procedure that enabled the school to deal 'quickly and effectively' with bullying and an accurate system for logging instances of bullying were recommended. A clear structure, lines of responsibility, guidance and advice for students, parents and teachers was also found to be important. Mediation and communication between the parents of the bully and the bullied could be facilitated by the school and clear messages about values and what is not acceptable should be introduced to students and parents, with one participant suggesting 'a year 6 open evening to introduce how the school deals with bullying and what the school values are'.

Parents engagement in the programme

The training included exploration of how parents could be involved in combating bullying in school. There was a general agreement that parents should be told about their child being bullied, preferably by the child. Some of the overall discussion focused on emotional support, with parents being able to listen, empathise and to show understanding and concern (such as regularly asking how the child is). Parents and families were seen as having a protective role through making the bullied individual feel safe, cared for and comfortable at home, with parent-child bonding sessions seen as being helpful. Some suggested that the child's friends and/or other families with experience with having a bullied child could support parents and families to deal with bullying. Other suggestions included practical interventions and problem solving, such as encouraging the child to report the bullying or reporting on behalf of the child if they are unable to do so themselves; meetings between the child, parent and tutors; negotiating a move to a different class or even a different school.

Parents identified some of the problems that are often encountered if their child is bullied in school. They said they can often feel helpless because they do not know who to contact at the school or how to notify the school of the bullying. Some of the parents also talked about the frustration of feeling ignored and not listened to by the school. Frustration could sometimes be taken out on the child or expressed through arguments with the bully's parents. However, there were also some positive suggestions of how parents can support their child if they are being bullied, particularly 'calming your child down' in order to 'listen empathically and understand the situation from the child's point of view'.

There was strong agreement that parents should be involved in combating bullying in the school by being enabled to 'have a voice'. Again, clarity and communication (including meetings and action plans) were cited by participants as being crucial for schools and parents to work together on instances of bullying. They felt that 'there should be a good, simple, clear school policy about bullying which is quick and effective in dealing with the bully including reasonable punishment' and that 'there should be meetings where parents, children and teachers get together to combat bullying with ongoing support'. Training on bullying was also seen as important.

Moving forward – recommendations from the workshops

As a result of joint action planning, several approaches and strategies were suggested as ways for schools and families to address bullying together. Communication and meetings between parents and teachers or the school were seen as vital and it was recognised that parental involvement with the school on issues of bullying was important. It was suggested that parents should be able to meet teachers to discuss concerns about bullying; teachers should communicate with and update parents about how the bullying of their child is being tackled (or progress on combating bullying in general) through phone calls, text or emails; termly parents' evenings should include discussion of any bullying issues; parent support groups could be set up for peer support and learning. It was recommended that the school create an online support resource for bullied students to speak up and share their thoughts on what should be done. The need for the school to support parental training and awareness raising was highlighted, with suggestions for workshops on the causes and effects of bullying and activity days so children can bond with their parents. More generally, there was a call for 'more security of social media' and a 'block on social networks' to reduce the instances of cyberbullying. It was also felt important that the school took responsibility for engaging with the parents of any child involved in bullying to give support.

Conclusion

This chapter drew on some of the findings from a large European project to illustrate how there is a need for much closer collaboration, communication and engagement across those working with situations involving homophobic/transphobic bullying. We have shared some of the key findings emerging from a review of the education policy literature on homophobic and transphobic bullying in the UK and used this to foreground a practice example case study led by the English project team. This developed and piloted a family and student led intervention within two secondary schools aimed at preventing homophobic and transphobic bullying. Whilst the approach of the family intervention in RAINBOW-HAS hardly touched some of these broader context issues, it was successful as a model in which to combine the contribution of parents, children at the school who may themselves have been subject to homophobic bullying, and the teachers at the school and was inclusive of all families. Although not formally evaluated, a description of the outcomes has provided some good insights into the issues common to young people in schools and generated some ideas for the school to work on based on local partnership and engagement. There is an urgent need to actively create meaningful networks which engage families and their children from all backgrounds to share the responsibility of protecting rights, taking on commitments, handling bullying, promoting support programmes, and generating positive cultures, conditions and reliable mechanisms for children and families at risk.

It was noticeable from our experience conducting RAINBOW-HAS that social work and related professionals have yet to tangibly enter these debates with significance. Social work has an intimate relationship with 'the family', since many aspects of practice are concerned with family life and problems, and exerts powerful claims about its interventions (Hicks, 2011). Social work has much less to do with mainstream education even though research evidence suggests that bullying involving homophobic and transphobic abuse is itself mainstream (Mishna et al., 2009) but it could and should have a role. Cocker (2015) reminds us that some of the more obvious differences are their coming out experiences and the effect this may have on extended family support and their different family gender constructs. These will manifest themselves in relation to a family's particular experiences living within their particular local community, the way in which they are able to engage with educational institutions and the impact of homophobic and transphobic bullying for both them and LGBT young people. RAINBOW-HAS has implications for social work with LGBT families as well as LGBT youth as there may be a complicated picture on the ground. Social workers have been shown to think uncritically about heteronormativity in their approach to assessment with families and young people (Hicks, 2011; Brown and Cocker, 2011; Cocker, 2015) and as we will see in our concluding chapter, social work knowledge and skills in this area tend to promote culturally competent models – an 'add-on' model for mastering knowledge of sexual difference. Whilst social work with LGBT families have changed markedly following extensive legislation regarding the age of consent, civil relationship recognition, marriage, and access to public goods and services, this new-found 'equality' in the diversity of ways in which we understand 'family' and family structures remains unsophisticated from a social work perspective (see Cocker, 2015). This is because societal discourses about families are firmly entrenched within a heteronormative framework, and this is enacted both within the social work and education communities. Combined with social work's relative silence on LGBT issues within its equality, diversity and human rights concerns (Cocker and Hafford-Letchfield, 2010, 2014), we suggest that there are implications for social work to respond in new and different ways, particularly given its role in service integration and systemic approaches to promoting children's well-being.

Strategies to address bullying require interventions at various levels within the system. This includes the need for deconstruction of traditional or dominant accounts of family life, which supports the increased visibility of sexuality within all institutions and acknowledges the complexity of managing identities. It also requires a transfer of power from professionals to service users and their communities so they can take more control and exercise choice in the way services support them to live their lives, and an appreciation of the values, connections and desires that bind LGBT social networks together so that there are parallel supports in legal, policy and service developments. Our practice example in RAINBOW-HAS demonstrates the value of engaging families in a wider debate around bullying that engages with policy and guidance, and recognises the value of tackling homophobic and transphobic bullying to ensure that families have the opportunities to connect around the same concerns for all of their children.

Key recommendations for applying research to professional practice

• Include topics on LGBT families in professional education and move away from fixed identities towards engaging with the more complex, multiple and fluid identities of LGBT people, reflecting their individuality and their social and economic context including education.

- Ensuring that we think critically about some of the problems that young people present with in social work services to identify homophobic and transphobic bullying issues and be ready to respond and support.
- Promoting LGBT advocacy and rights based interventions in work with LGBT populations
- Developing partnership with schools to support them with young people experiencing bullying issues.

Acknowledgements

RAINBOW-HAS was co-funded by the European Union's Fundamental Rights and Citizenship programme. The authors thank the partner membership organisations and especially all of the parents, carers, families, schools and young people and their advocates who participated in this research and who made it possible.

Special thanks to the parents, teachers and young people who took part in this project.

References

Adams, N., Cox, T., Dunstan, L. (2004) I am the hate that dare not speak its name. Dealing with homophobia in secondary Schools. *Educational Psychology in Practice*, 20 (3), 259–269.

Amnesty International (2014) *Yogyakarta Principles: The Application of International Human Rights Law in Relation to Sexual Orientation and Gender Identity.* London, Amnesty International.

Ararteko (2015) *Rights through Alliances: Innovating and Networking both within Homes and Schools. Project Report.* Milan, Ararteko.

Birkett, M., Espelage, D.L., Koenig, B. (2009) LGB and questioning students in schools: The moderating effects of homophobic bullying and school climate on negative outcomes. *Journal of Youth and Adolescence*, 38 (7), 989–1000.

British Psychological Society (2014) *Safeguarding and Promoting the Welfare of Children Position Paper.* Leicester, The British Psychological Society.

Brown, H.C., Cocker, C. (2011) *Social Work with Lesbians & Gay Men*, London, Sage.

Cocker, C. (2015) 'Social work and adoption: The impact of civil partnership and same sex marriage. In N. Barker and D. Monk (eds.) *From Civil Partnership to Same Sex Marriage: Interdisciplinary Reflections.* Abingdon, Routledge. pp. 97–114.

Cocker, C., Hafford-Letchfield, T. (2010) Critical commentary: Out and proud? Social work's relationship with Lesbian and gay equality. *British Journal of Social Work*, 40 (6), 1996–2008.

Cocker, C., Hafford-Letchfield, T. (2014) (Eds) *Rethinking anti-discriminatory practice and anti-oppressive theories for social work practice*, Basingstoke, Palgrave. pp. 263, ISBN 9781137023971

Cocker, C., Hafford-Letchfield, T., Ryan, P., Baron, C. (2018) Positioning discourse on homophobia in schools: What have lesbian and gay families got to say? *Qualitative Social Work*. [Online first]

DePalma, R., Atkinson, E. (2009) 'No Outsiders': Moving beyond a discourse of tolerance to challenge heteronormativity in primary schools. *British Educational Research Journal*, 35 (6), 837–855.

Department for Children, Education and Schools (2004) *The Charter for Action (Department for Education and Skills).* London, HMSO.

Department for Education and Skills (2005). *Bullying: Don't Suffer in Silence.* London: DfES Publications.

DCSF (2007) *Safe to Learn: Embedding Anti-Bullying Work in Schools – Preventing and Responding to Homophobic Bullying in Schools.* London: DCSF.

Department for Education (2010) *The Importance of Teaching White Paper 2010 Prevention of Bullying.* London, The Stationary Office.

Department for Education (2013) *Preventing and Tackling Bullying: Advice for Head-teachers, Staff and Governing Bodies.* London, Department for Education.

Department for Education and Skills (2000) *Bullying: Don't Suffer in Silence.* London, HMSO.

Department for Education and Skills (2003a) *Anti-Bullying Charter for Action.* London, HMSO.

Department for Education and Skills (2003b) *Every Child Matters.* London, HMSO.

EU (2000) Charter of Fundamental Rights of the European Union (2000/C 364/01). *Journal of the European Communities.* Strasbourg, The European Union.

EU (2012) *Treaty on European Union and the Treaty on the Functioning of the European Union 2012/C 326/01.* Strasbourg, European Union.

EU (2012) *Consolidated versions of the Treaty on European Union and the Treaty on the Functioning of the European Union 2012/C 326/* Strasburg, Euro-Lex.

Farrington, D.P., Ttofi, M.M. (2010) *School Based Programs to Reduce Bullying and Victimization.* Oslo, Campbell Systematic Review.

Guasp, A. (2010) *Different Families: The Experiences of Children with Lesbian and Gay Parents.* London, Stonewall.

Hafford-Letchfield, T., Cocker, C., Ryan, P. (2016) Rights through Alliances: Findings from a European project tackling homophobic and transphobic bullying in schools through the engagement of families and young people. *British Journal of Social Work*, 6 (8), 2338–2356.

Hicks, S. (2011) *Lesbian, Gay and Queer Parenting: Families, Intimacies, Genealogies.* Basingstoke, Palgrave.

HMG (1998) *School Standards and Framework Act, Chp 31.* London, The Stationary Office.

HMG (2010) *Equality Act 2010.* London, The Stationary Office.

House of Commons Education and Skills Committee (2007) *Bullying: Third Report of Session 2006–07.* London, The Stationery Office.

Hunt, R., Jensen, J. (2007) *The School Report: The Experiences of Young Gay People in Britain's Schools.* London, Stonewall.

ILGA-Europe (2015) *Annual Review of the Human Rights Situation of Lesbian, Gay, Bisexual, Trans and Intersex People in Europe.* Belgium, ILGA-Europe.

McDermott, E. (2010) *Researching and Monitoring Adolescence and Sexual Orientation: Asking the Right Questions at the Right Time.* London, Equality and Human Rights Commission.

Mishna, F., Newman, P., Daley, A., Solomon, S. (2009) Bullying of lesbian and gay youth: A qualitative investigation. *British Journal of Social Work*, 39 (8), 1598–1614.

Monk, D. (2009) Challenging homophobic bullying in schools: The politics of progress. *International Journal of Law in Context*, 7 (2), 181–207.

National Union of Teachers (2017) *Working for a Fairer Future: Advice for Members on LGBT Equality in Education with Guidance for School Representatives*. London, NUT.

Ofsted (2002). *Report on sex and relationships*. Retrieved from www.OFSTED.gov.uk/public/docs02/sexandrelationships.pdf.

Ofsted (2012) *Tackling Homophobic Bullying and Ingrained Attitudes at School*. London, Ofsted.

Rivers, I. (2001) The bullying of sexual minorities at school: Its nature and long-term correlates. *Educational and Child Psychology*, 18 (1), 32–46.

Shepherd, J., Learner, S. (2010) Lessons on gay history cut homophobic bullying in north London school. *The Guardian*, 25/10/2010.

Smith, P.K., Kupferberg, A., Mora-Merchan, J.A., Samara, M., Bosley, S., Osborn, R. (2012) A content analysis of school anti-bullying policies: A follow-up after six years, *Educational Psychology in Practice*, 28 (1), 47–70.

Stonewall (2017) *School Report: The Experiences of Lesbian, Gay, Bi and Trans Young People in Britain's Schools in 2017*. London, Stonewall and University of Cambridge.

Tippett, N., Houlston, C., Smith, P.K. (2010) *Prevention and Response to Identity-Based Bullying among Local Authorities in England, Scotland and Wales*, London, Equality and Human Rights Commission.

UNESCO (2012) *Education Sector Responses to Homophobic Bullying: Booklet 8*, Paris, France, United Nations Educational, Science and Cultural Organisation.

Walton, G. (2006), H-cubed: A primer on bullying and sexuality diversity for educators. *Professional Development Perspectives*, 6 (2), 13–20.

4   Intimacy in young women's friendships

Symbols and rituals

Katie Letchfield and Trish Hafford-Letchfield

Introduction

The phenomenon of friendship and its function and purpose within social work and social care is significantly under-researched. This chapter outlines the function of symbols and ritual in relation to ideals of 'friendships' among young women. It draws principally from a small qualitative study involving semi-structured interviews with five women aged 18–25 years during which they discussed their friendships. We discuss key themes from the data analysis and draw out the importance of intimacy in friendships for young women within this stage of the life course. The findings indicated that not only do rituals and symbols create and support internal intimacy, but also constituted practices informed by a cultural ideal of what it means to be a 'friend'. The implications for how social work assessment and interventions takes these into account when working with young people and other service user groups is then explored.

Theoretical perspectives on 'friendships'

The term 'friend' or 'friendship' is inherently problematic (see Allan, 1979; Pahl, 2000; Spencer and Pahl, 2006) with idealised voluntarism and non-beneficial characteristics (Spencer and Pahl, 2006). Friendship has been described as the archetype of a 'pure relationship' (Giddens, 1991:6); one that is entered into freely and exists for the sole purpose of whatever rewards the relationship can deliver. It may also be based on reciprocity if there is an exchange of goods or help. The assumption that friendships are always a positive experience has also been questioned (Davies, 2011; Smart et al., 2012). Smart et al.'s (2012) study found that women were more likely than men to persevere with 'difficult' friendships. Women were found to have 'a strong moral regime of friendship', which meant they were unable to abandon friends even when the friendship became a chore (p. 96). Spencer and Pahl (2006) identified eight categories of friendship ranging from 'associate' (someone who shares a common activity or interest) to 'soul mate' which they identify as the most multifaceted type of friendship (p. 69). 'Soul mate' friendships involve opportunities for confiding, providing emotional support, helping each other out and enjoying each other's company. 'Soul mate' friends may feel they have a similar outlook on life, and the friendship is characterised by a high level of commitment and a strong sense of intimacy. The study reported here focuses on this latter category of friendship. The literature also suggests that the more complex the relationship becomes the more there is a sense of trust and intimacy and that high levels of intimacy are found to correspond positively with ritual enactment (Bruess and Pearson, 1997; Smart et al., 2012).

Gender differences are highlighted in the literature, including same-sex friendships. Hook et al. (2003) suggest that women are more likely to be socialised into forming and valuing close relationships. Their study found that women tried to create and maintain intimacy through talking and discussion, whereas men utilised activities and 'doing' (p. 465). Tannen (1990) looked at male and female conversations from a sociolinguistic standpoint, and described more 'rapport talk' (the elaboration on why and how) between women whilst men tend more towards 'report talk'. These 'why' and 'how' function of rituals and symbols formed the focus of interest in this study of young women's same-gender friendships. We have also incorporated the concept of 'doing' (Morgan, 1996, 2011) and 'display' (Finch, 2007) into our current understanding of rituals and symbols. Whereas existing literature tends to focus on the internality of ritual/symbol function, by integrating theories of 'doing' and 'display', there is greater potential to increase the depth of analysis of this phenomenon, particularly in relation to the externality as well as internality of ritual and symbol functions.

Relevance of friendships for social work and social care

The individual nature of friendship differentiates it from other types of relationships, such as colleagues or other formal role positions, because friends cannot be substituted or interchanged and may be entered into for the pure enjoyment of interaction and other non-instrumental reasons (Allan, 1979:42). Colleagues or family members may also be 'friends', for example, siblings describing one another as one's closest 'soul mate' (Spencer and Pahl, 2006:33). However, differences in these relationships include the exercise of free choice that allows interaction to go beyond prescribed organisational or familial affiliations (Allan, 1979). When thinking about social work and social care, these dynamics come into play in relation to identifying and valuing people in somebody's support and care networks and being aware of any nuances in the nature of relationships where there may be dependency. Further, our interventions have the potential to disrupt or challenge the making and sustaining of friendships and thus impact on young women's well-being at a time of crisis as well as longer term. Friendships may also be instrumental in bridging gaps in support and services not otherwise provided (Galupo et al., 2014).

The implicit assumption that friendships are a positive experience also belies that they may also involve a sense of guilt and obligation, especially in more complex relationships such as 'soul mate' friendships (Smart et al., 2012). The termination of 'difficult' friendships is much harder and there a range of examples in the safeguarding literature, for example, the rise of 'mate crime' in the experiences of people with learning disabilities (Landman, 2014) and the exploitation of vulnerable older people (Crosby et al., 2008). In their study of the friendship networks of homeless people with problematic use of drugs and alcohol, Neal and Brown (2016) found eight categories of friends emerged from their data, with family-like friends appearing to offer the most constant practical and emotional support. Yet the environment within homeless hostels operated strict rules and policies which banned visitors or imposed curfews, which can undermine relationships and create tensions and mistrust between individuals (Stevenson, 2013). Weeks et al. (2001) identified the increased importance of friendships for people in gender and sexual minority communities. Friendships were found to buffer people from the social isolation or rejection associated with homophobia and transphobia, and friendships were emphasised during times of social change, which is particularly salient when an individual's identity is at odds with social norms (Galupo et al., 2014).

Rituals and symbols in friendships

The study reported here explored the role of rituals and symbols in the friendships of young women and attempted to bridge a theoretical gap on friendship rituals from other areas of literature on personal life. Rituals are 'behaviour [that is] jointly enacted and shared by relational partners' (Pearson et al., 2010:465) while symbols are 'markers of group identity' (Collins, 2005:36). Both can be seen as ways to communicate identity (Suter et al., 2008:30). Baxter (1987) argued that symbols are statements about the relationship that communicate its level of intimacy and solidarity. Rituals and symbols can be identified by two components; a 'textual' meaning (physical characteristics of the symbol/actual behaviour of the ritual) and a 'social' meaning (the unique meaning that artefact/behaviour takes on to the people in the relationship) (Pearson et al., 2010:465). The significance attributed to these behaviours through repetitive enactment helps our understanding of how everyday practices become ritualised, and how passive artefacts become symbolic. The type of intimacy found in familial and committed romantic relationships is often mirrored in 'soul mate' friendships (Hook et al., 2003) making it reasonable to deduce that many types of rituals and symbols found in studies on familial/romantic relationships may also be present in 'soul mate' friendships. The study described here has therefore mainly drawn on research done on romantic or familial rituals and symbols, though attempts are made to highlight when and where differences will occur.

Rituals have two distinguishing features: routine behaviour and the associated meaning for that behaviour. Bruess and Pearson's study consisted of semi-structured interviews that probed the nature of rituals that couples/ friends enact or had enacted in the past. They identified five different types of rituals: social/fellowship, idiosyncratic/symbolic, communication rituals, share/support/vent, task/favours.

Baxter's study on friendship **symbols** (1987) highlights the importance of their 'textual' meaning (physical characteristics and how they may be interpreted to people outside of the friendship) and their 'social' meaning (the unique meaning it takes on to the people in the relationship). She argues that no two relationship symbols are the same, but they can be linked or categorised, and has identified five distinct categories: physical objects, cultural artefacts, special places, special events or times and behavioural artefacts. Bell and Healy (1992) argue that friendships also develop 'personalised codes' or linguistic symbols, which may develop naturally over time or form specifically to deal with certain situations.

Further within the literature there appears to be two different types of functions of rituals and symbols, their internal and the external functions. The internal function is concerned with the individuals involved in a friendship and the external function is concerned with people outside of the relationship. Rituals and symbols are a way for participants in a friendship to create a unique friendship. Symbols are statements about the relationship that communicate the level of intimacy and solidarity. Secret symbols, particularly language codes, shut other people out of the relationship and 'establish a boundary' (Betcher, 1987:48). Baxter (1987) identified many uses for symbols in relationships, such as linking the past to the present, allowing the relationship to withstand periods of change. In their study, Bell and Healy (1992) found support for their hypothesis that increased idiom use in a friendship would be positively correlated with the perceived intimacy.

Bruess and Pearson (1997) argue that rituals 'create a historically significant shared sense of the relationship' (p. 26), which help to provide a sense of stability and normality during periods of change. From the perspective of those who enact them, Pearson et al.'s study (2010) showed that couples with a higher number of rituals also had a higher level of perceived intimacy. This was attributed to rituals providing the opportunity to be emotionally close, and as individuals participate in being open with each other the perceived intimacy of the relationship is increased. Rituals can be ways in which individuals 'do' or perform relationships. 'Doing' relationships facilitate the creation of identity through the completion of mundane or ordinary tasks on a regular basis (Suter et al., 2008:38). Further, Morgan's (1996) work on 'doing' family shows the ways in which an identity of a family emerges through family practices which need to be sustained in order for the family's identity to be sustained. In Suter et al.'s study, the identity created was that of a mother and a lesbian, however it is more than feasible that the identity of 'friend' can also be created by 'doing' friendship.

Study design and methods

This qualitative study aimed to study friendship through symbolic inter-actionism and how these interactions help individuals to negotiate their friendships. The research questions were:

1 In what ways do different categories of rituals add to the perceived inti-macy of the friendship?
2 In what ways do different categories of symbols add to the perceived intimacy of the friendship?
3 How important is 'displaying' these rituals/symbols to outsiders for the participants in order to legitimise the friendship?

Snowball sampling was used to recruit five women in the target age group 18–25 willing to discuss their personal friendships. Details of the partici-pants are shown in Table 4.1.

Semi-structured interviews lasting approximately 60 minutes were used to explore participants' personal friendships. An inductive approach (Bryman, 2008) posited questions such as: What did you do the last time you saw each other? Do you usually do that? Do you have any special phrases or language you only use with each other? Questions permitted 'travel' with respond-ents down avenues of thought that spontaneously appeared (Best, 2012:78). For example, the first question 'tell me about the friend you have chosen, who are they?' evoked some responses as simple as 'I've chosen Fiona who I live with now and have known for three years'. Sometimes it also yielded data in the first very first instance such as 'it's my friend K… well we always used to walk to school together'. The term 'always' and 'used to' were ver-bal signifiers that some kind of ritual or symbol may have been identified. Thus these were then probed immediately, rather than being bound to a set list of questions. To ensure that participants were able to participate fully, the terms 'rituals' and 'symbols' were avoided as much as possible.

The interviews were digitally recorded and transcribed. Ethical ap-proval was granted by Manchester University. Data analysis drew on a framework constructed around four of the five types of rituals identi-fied by Bruess and Pearson (1997); types of symbols identified by Baxter

Table 4.1 Characteristics of sample

Pseudonym	Age	Profession	Length of friendship being discussed (years)
Rachel	22	Student	3
Jordanne	23	Teaching assistant	3
Michelle	19	Au pair	10
Faye	22	Student	17
Scarlett	23	Office manager	9

Table 4.2 Characteristics of rituals and symbols from the data

1	*Social ritual*: Rituals that involve enjoyable activities and socialising.	
2	*Idiosyncratic ritual*: Rituals that are unique to that friendship such as play rituals or celebration rituals.	
3	*Communication ritual*: Rituals that support regular communication such as phone calls or emails.	
4	*Share/support/vent ritual*: Rituals that support emotional sharing.	
5	*Tasks/favours ritual*: Rituals that involve doing something for or with a friend.	
6	*Physical symbol*: Physical objects such as gifts, photographs etc.	
7	*Cultural artefacts*: Symbol Intangible symbols such as favourite song, shared culture or genre.	
8	*Special places*: Symbol Places with significant meaning.	
9	*Special times/events*: Symbol Times of the day/week/month/year with significant meaning.	
10	*Personalised codes*: Symbol Nicknames, special words, language patterns.	

(1987) and the concept of 'personalised codes' identified by Bell and Healy (1997). Table 4.2 shows the broad categories used to code the interview data.

Interpretation using these frameworks occurred on many levels; from the primary experience of the ritual/symbol by respondents, to their telling of it, including how the researcher related to the experience, analysed and presented it (Miller and Glassner, 2011:134). Embedded in this approach is the notion that the interview itself was a form of symbolic interaction; where respondents and the researcher constructed a narrative about the social world (Miller and Glassner, 2011:132). Many questions had emphasis on the respondents' subjectivity, for example, 'how do you think that affected your friendship?' rather than 'how did that affect your friendship?'

Transcripts were searched for 'central themes' (Best, 2012:85), following the colour coding of rituals, symbols, internal functions and external functions no matter how trivial. All possible rituals and symbols were then listed separately for each respondent, and sorted into the ten categories noted in Table 4.2. Transcripts were further coded along the lines of 'internal functions' and 'external functions'. Secondary analysis involved going back to the lists of rituals and symbols and eliminating any that did not fit the definition entirely. For example, Rachel acknowledged, 'always going to the club together' which in the initial analysis was identified as a ritual. During secondary analysis, this 'routine behaviour' appeared to have no 'associated meaning' (Pearson et al., 2010:465), and was therefore decoded as a ritual in the final analyses. This introduced an element of subjectivity in the analysis but was necessary within the limitations of this study. This transparency should be acknowledged to appreciate the validity of the findings within this context.

The remainder of this chapter discusses the findings from the study within three key themes.

Findings

Rituals

Seventy-six rituals were identified, averaging 15.2 rituals per respondent. All five categories of rituals (social, idiosyncratic, communication, tasks/favours, share/support/vent) were identified. Most were enacted regularly but a few were behaviours respondents 'used to do'. Rituals were used to both create and sustain intimacy. Physical 'enacted behaviours' more often than not did not involve talking; however, the reason most rituals existed were to facilitate the start of some type of discussion. Exceptions involved task/favour rituals, enacted when a seemingly boring or mundane task required completion. However, even in this category, the women occasionally identified that the main reason the friend was enlisted was to create opportunity for talking. This echoes Hook et al.'s (2003) claim that talking is preferred way in which women try to create intimacy.

Creating intimacy

Although share/support/vent rituals were the least frequently occurring, (six identified), these were vital in the creation of intimacy and supported emotional sharing between friends or signified a 'heart-to-heart' discussion. Rachel, for example, identified always playing a certain song, 'His Eye Is on the Sparrow', when her friend is upset. The effect was two-fold; first it immediately makes her friend laugh which releases tension and lightens the mood. Second and more importantly, it signifies Rachel's availability for emotional support and discussion. This example also highlights the intrinsic link between ritual and symbol, thus making the two phenomena inseparable (see Durkheim, 1918:231). In this example, the symbol (the song) became an integral part of the behaviour enactment and would have lost significance if a different song were used in the same situation. Similarly, if the song were played in a different setting it would take on a different meaning.

Share/support/vent rituals incited an encouraging reception and were perceived to be a positive occurrence; indicating a level of intimacy and trust in the friendship. Share/support/vent rituals allowed respondents and their friends to be both physically and emotionally close, which in turn increased the perceived intimacy (Pearson et al., 2010). Further, a 'heart-to-heart' needed to happen more than once, and be regular and ritualised because that's what 'keeps [the friendship] going'.

Idiosyncratic rituals were the second most occurring category, with 14 rituals identified. This ritual was often borne out of a single past event, enjoyable and so repeated until it took on ritualised characteristics. Bruess and Pearson (1997) comment that idiosyncratic rituals often represent some kind of aspect of the couple's relational history. This was evident in Jordanne's account of herself and her friend having a special dance move; 'the hula hoop', displayed to each other any time music was played, such as in a club.

> I feel like, hahaha that's so funny... it probably reminds you of why you're close to that person. Coz you're thinking, oh yeah I remember that shared experience and it was really funny. It probably reinforces in my mind that she's a fun person, we have the same sense of humour, things like that.

A shared sense of humour is known to be one of the most important aspects of friendship (Spencer and Pahl, 2006). Further, this sense of shared history supports friendships during periods of instability or change. Faye recalled her friend getting a video camera at age eight or nine for Christmas, and together making a Celine Dion music video. Making performance videos is now a regular behaviour for the friendship:

> FAYE: 'Every time we're together she finds this song, and then we just make up these most ridiculous videos. Like these dance videos. We've been doing that for years. Like years.... From when we were really young and she still has this obsession with making these dance videos so every time we're together we'll do something that involves... making something up and recording it.'

The context of friendships is also important because Faye may not physically see her friend for months at a time as employment took her to another country. More so than other respondents who saw their friends more regularly, Faye's idiosyncratic rituals highlight the 'shared history' (Bruess and Pearson, 1997:35) and reinforced their closeness to each other when they met again.

Maintaining intimacy

The maintenance of a high level of intimacy was of paramount importance. Social rituals existed to support (rather than create) high levels of intimacy within these 'soul mate' friendships. Thirty-two rituals were identified in this category. Social rituals involved activities done recreationally and for pleasure, for example, regularly baking together or watching a certain TV show. These seemingly normal and everyday activities were attributed with personal meaning that distinguished them as rituals, rather than general everyday activities. Faye noted how she and her friend usually did activities inside rather than outside, and describes what 'usually' happens when they spend time together:

We have an obsession with things like E-Television; together that's our thing. Like 'The Kardashians' or 'Chelsea Lately' and stuff, so like we'd like be all night watching things like that. That's our thing... it's just like a blanket and something really crappy on TV.

The phrase 'our thing' is used twice within this short quote, so clearly this behaviour has 'associated meaning' for Faye (Pearson et al., 2010:465). Further, whilst watching 'crappy' TV may be an activity undertaken by many people, when probed, Faye noted that she only shared this activity with that particular friend; never on her own or with other people. Thus, both components of a ritual, the 'enacted behaviour' and the 'associated meaning', were present.

The 'doing together' of these activities provided an opportunity to talk, fulfilling the main aim of rituals in this category. Share/support/vent rituals supported deep and emotional 'heart-to-hearts', but social rituals supported 'catching-up' and general discussions. Rachel describes types of conversations during her social rituals as 'just talking rubbish really', whilst Michelle expresses them as 'very light hearted'. Further humour was important in these types of discussions (in comparison to 'heart-to-hearts'). Michelle notes:

Yeah we talk... the funnier the better basically... anything to make you giggle.

Bruess and Pearson (1997) argue that social rituals are important in maintaining friendships. Even seemingly trivial and 'nothing'-ness rituals attribute to the maintenance of intimacy, through spending time together and keeping in touch (p. 38). Their significance cannot be overlooked, nor the function of mundane conversations trivialised. Twelve communication rituals were identified for keeping in touch, and all respondents reported making an effort to communicate with their friend regularly, emphasising the high use of technology (phoning monthly, Skyping weekly, and texting/WhatsApping daily). When questioned about these efforts, Scarlett responded:

Just to touch base with each other. To find out what's been going on. Yeah I guess that's what you do with friend's right?

Like social rituals, communication rituals provide the platform for discussion. However, where the function of social rituals can be subtle, or less explicit than 'doing' activities (such as baking), communication rituals are obvious in their purpose. Bruess and Pearson (1997) assert that communication rituals are common among friends, and can help to sustain friendships during periods of change (p. 39). Scarlett, who had the longest friendship in length (19 years), noted that she and her friend 'had been through a lot... first boyfriends, moving away from home, serious illness... going away to college and uni'. Communicating on a regular basis meant her friend was 'not going anywhere', thus Scarlett felt she could 'rely on her in a different way [from her other friends]'.

'Doing' friendship

All categories of rituals supported the 'doing' of friendship. Respondents enacted these rituals as ways of confirming their identity as a 'friend'. Smart el al. (2012) found that friendship can generate feelings of obligation and expectation, as echoed here. However, whilst Smart et al. focused on how feelings of obligation are experienced in a negative way, feelings of obligation were both a positive and a negative aspect of friendship. This is best illustrated by looking at examples of tasks/favour rituals.

Twelve tasks/favour rituals were identified, including examples where the women had to complete a mundane or non-enjoyable task, and where doing this with a friend made the activity seem more enjoyable. These examples reinforced the desire for talking opportunities, as discussed earlier. 'Doing' friendship was seen in the second subcategory of tasks/favour rituals, which involved doing favours for the respondent's friend, without any material reward. Examples included frequently 'doing her [friend's] roots' or giving lifts in the car. Jordanne's reasons for this were:

> Maybe it's like that feeling of having a duty to someone. And maybe that's about feeling we're in this together, I can get you this… it reinforces that you like them enough to do that.

Rachel responded:

> I think it would be returned in some way or another at some point eventually… I think its just part of the friendship… she'd do it for me.

For both Jordanne and Rachel, the sense of obligation is not a negative aspect of friendship, but a way of proving to themselves and to their friend that they are able to fulfil a selfless and altruistic role of 'friend'. For Rachel, favours were part and parcel of what friendship involves; neither positive nor negative emphasising perceived reciprocity which Allan (1979) maintains as a key characteristic of friendship. Smart et al. (2012) observed that feelings of obligation can also be experienced in negative ways. Scarlett stated that even though they had been friends a long time, sometimes her friendship could be quite difficult. When asked if she ever did favours for her friend she replied:

> Not so much physically. I guess sometimes she… it sounds really bad, but she complains a lot about things. So she wants my time and opinions on things that I don't necessarily think are that important.

Here the sense of obligation to discuss issues with her friend was perceived as a chore. When probed further about why she allowed herself to be pressed, she replied:

> Just to be supportive. Coz it was important to her. And I just think, I wouldn't like it if something really mattered to me [she was like] well I don't care I don't want to talk about it. That's kind of selfish.

For Scarlett, the sense of reciprocity involved expectations of a similar behaviour from her friend in the reverse situation and a sense of obligation; to not be 'selfish', the antithesis to being a friend. Although focused on tasks/favour rituals specifically here, it was noted that for all respondents, the completion of rituals in any category constitutes practices of 'doing' friendship by sustaining practices that are socially associated with friendship (Morgan, 1996).

Symbols

Seventy-six symbols were identified in this study, with an average of 15.2 symbols per respondent. All five categories of symbols (physical, cultural artefact, special time/event, special place, personalised code) were identified and sustained the friendships in many ways. They provided feelings of comfort, they highlighted the uniqueness of the friendship and they created boundaries between the friends and the outside world. Symbols are often a result of ritualised behaviour (Collins, 2005:36), therefore many symbols were also linked to a certain ritual. However, where rituals are an active and conscious way for the respondents to maintain friendship solidarity, symbols demonstrated that this maintenance had happened.

Symbols provide the function of reminding respondents that they were engaged in an intimate friendship and gave a feeling of comfort, with physical symbols being the most obvious examples. Physical symbols were the third most frequently occurring symbol, with 14 symbols identified. Many included gifts given by their friends and pictures of them together. Michelle took a little wooden 'love spoon', given to her by her friend, to France when she moved there:

> I don't know (why), I just like it, it's nice to have a piece of home and a piece of her.

The love spoon represents a physical manifestation of the intimacy Michelle experiences with her friend and provides comfort and a sense of familiarity in a foreign place; thus 'bridging a transition between the familiar past and forces of novelty and change' (Baxter, 1987:263). This is similar to the way in which rituals also help friendships to withstand periods of change. The 'love spoon', like many other physical symbols, was seen to provide a 'certainty about the relationship' due to its tangible properties (Baxter, 1987:263).

Photographs also provided an important physical source of comfort and all respondents recounted being together in photos even if not displayed:

> It's a good memory, of second year. That is just one instance of being in a club but it makes me think of all the times we've been out and had fun nights.

Baxter (1987) argues that symbols provide 'concrete metacommunicating statements about the abstract qualities of [friendship]' (p. 263), and Jordanne notes that photographs remind her of the good memories her and her friend share. Special time/event symbols were also seen to provide a sense of familiarity within the friendship. Special time/event symbols were the fourth most frequently occurring symbol, with five symbols identified. These represented a special day or period in their life reminiscent of their friend which provided comfort when the friend was absent.

Highlighting the uniqueness of the friendship

A function of symbols that emerged was the emphasis of the idiosyncratic characteristics of particular friendships. For example, personalised codes are ways in which respondents highlighted to themselves and to others the 'uniqueness' of the friendship (Bell et al., 1987:50). Personalised codes were the most frequently occurring symbol, with 37 symbols identified. Within personalised codes, nicknames (both for themselves and for other people) were the most common type of symbol, with examples including Voldemort, Farm Girl, Handsome Man, Airey Fairy and The Overgrown Baby. Phrases or sayings were also identified within this category, examples including 'oooh that's a bit posh', 'I've squashed my banana' and 'where can I put my piano?'

  Personalised codes were used only within these specific friendships. Most were language based but not limited to linguistics. Non-verbal signals, i.e. body language or moves, were included in this category. Faye demonstrated a specific look that her and her friend always give each other if they do not like someone else:

> She'll pull that face and I'll know exactly what she means. She won't have to say anything I'll just know... and I'll pull it back, if I agree. I don't do that with anyone else.

A 'unique language' is cultivated, and it transmits the feelings and values of the friendship members (Bell et al., 1987:47–48). Therefore, one function of this personalised code is to show that Faye and her friend share something that no one else understands.

  Cultural artefacts served to highlight the uniqueness of the friendship and were the second most occurring category, with 16 symbols identified.

Scarlett acknowledged a shared Jamaican heritage where she and her friend were brought up on a 'similar kind of music' and understood references to 'typical Jamaican' aspects of their lives. The context is important because Scarlett went to a majority-white private school and being able to share with her friend knowledge about a certain culture meant that Scarlett regarded that friendship as unique.

Creating boundaries

It is argued that personalised codes help to establish boundaries between the outside world and the relationship, and that intimacy is maintained through this exclusion of outsiders (Baxter, 1987; Bell et al., 1987). This was supported to some extent in this study. Rachel and her friend always refer to an ex-boyfriend as 'Voldemort', a nickname chosen due to slight physical resemblance between the ex-boyfriend and the character from the 'Harry Potter' series. More importantly, this private verbal signifier to the other established who they were talking about to the exclusion of others:

> She never calls him by his real name, [if she referred to him by his real name]... that would be really strange. Coz not many people know about him and her, so it's like a code name so she can... so people don't know who she's talking about when she says something about him.

These linguistic symbols were used in both private and public settings, but in public functioned to maintain privacy when talking about a personal issue. Rachel gave the example of saying 'S.F.' instead of 'sexually frustrated':

> Now we can use that and people don't know what you're saying, coz you're not gonna walk around saying, oh I'm so sexually frustrated, you know? So if we're out shopping or something we'd say, oh I'm so S.F.

Other respondents stated similar nicknames, phrases or non-verbal signifiers used in public places to create a boundary between them and outsiders to the friendship. However, in 25 out of the 37 personalised codes identified, the women stated that there was nothing inherently private or personal about their idiomatic communication. Many respondents identified making an effort not to use personalised communication in front of other people because it felt rude and exclusionary. There were mixed findings of whether personalised codes were used to establish and maintain privacy.

Special places

The special places category did not yield much data and were the least frequently occurring symbol, with four symbols identified. These symbols were places where respondents and their friend frequented, and came to be associated with each other. In some instances, its function was to highlight the uniqueness of the friendship, for example, playing a certain genre of music in a nightclub that only they enjoyed or was exclusive to them. In other cases, these special places provided a sense of comfort and familiarity. Further study could be done on these types of symbols to provide a more definitive case for their function.

Doing friendship

There are two key components of Morgan's theory on 'doing' families in this study; the sense of the active, and the linking of history and biography (2011:7) were asserted with less focus on mundane and ordinary tasks. In four out of the five friendships investigated, time spent together was categorised by a sense of fun. Rituals can contribute to being 'active' in the friendship (Morgan, 2011:6). Morgan argues that families should be seen as 'doing' their relationships through seemingly trivial or meaningless tasks, which moves away from the idea of family as a static structure. Rituals in this sense added to a sense of actively 'doing' the relationship. When asked why Jordanne completed the task/favour ritual of routinely starting a new fad diet (inevitably given up within a few days) with her friend, she stated:

> [I do it]... to think, oh we're still doing things together... we're in this together.

Thus diets are always done together, never separately. This ritualised behaviour proves to Jordanne that she is active in the friendship, and that it is still alive. Jordanne is not only 'defined' herself as a friend, but can be seen to complete certain tasks in order to 'do' her role (Morgan, 2011:6).

'Displaying' friendship

Although respondents indicated a level of 'display' through physical symbols, particularly photographs, and the interview itself was a tool for 'display', the concept of 'display' should not be hastily applied to friendship rituals and symbols.

Within the category of displaying friendships through physical symbols, photographs were highly indicative of a degree of 'display' within the 'soul mate' friendships. When asked about having photographs on display of her and her friend, Scarlett said:

> Erm... I dunno, coz she's someone that I care about and I have other pictures of people that I care about, like close friends or family members. She's a special friend so I wanted to have a photo of her up.

Although a seemingly trivial detail, consider if Scarlett were to use the word 'and' in place of the word 'so'. 'So' implies a relationship between the displaying of a photograph and the level of 'special'ness of the friendship. Only 'special friends' deserve a place on the wall; that is how outsiders can gauge how important the friend is to Scarlett. Dermott and Seymour (2011) also conclude that 'displaying friendship' may be more necessary if the two people involved do not easily 'look' like friends from the outside. Although Faye and her friend were of the same ethnicity, gender and age, Faye said, 'me and her are quite different, and she's different to my other friends'.

Faye described a picture she has on display in her room of the two of them:

> It us when we were a lot younger and we both got these lilac shirts and these white trousers, and we both thought we were absolutely amazing. So we're standing in my kitchen doing the Spice Girls peace sign. And I remember on the day I was like, come on do the peace sign, and she was like, no I don't want to do the peace sign! [because she didn't like the Spice Girls]. And I just remember that showed how different we were, and it always makes me think that... So in the picture I'm really giving it the bit, the full throttle with the peace and the pouted lips and this whole Spice Girls thing, like proper Baby Spice. And she's fucking Grumpy Spice standing beside me. And that always stands out to me.

The photograph is telling of the character of the friendship; the differences between Faye and her friend are summed up. However, Faye stated that she wanted it up on her wall because

> ... because she is my best friend and obviously I want the most important people. At the time I think, I just remember being so proud that we were best friend, it was like, this is me and my best friend.

Faye uses the photograph to show that 'this is my [friendship] and it works' (see Finch, 2007:70). Similar views were expressed by other respondents within the physical symbol category, particularly in regard to photographs or gifts. We can conclude that these are indeed used as 'tools' that support the 'display' of these friendships (Finch, 2007:77).

'Displaying' in the interview

Another way of thinking about 'display' is by considering the interview itself as a 'display' of friendship, where respondents set out to show that through the use of rituals and symbols, they were in fact 'soul mate' friends. Finch argues narratives are 'tools for display' (2007:77) whilst Weeks et al. (2011) also comment that 'through narratives individuals... affirm their identities and present relationships as viable and valid' (p. 11). The narratives about rituals and symbols told throughout the interviews provided ways for respondents to communicate 'their friendship' and its character.

Rituals seemed to provide a positive experience for respondents; many of which are characterised by a sense of fun, particularly idiosyncratic rituals almost exclusively done to provoke the shared experience of laughing. As fun is an important characteristic of friendship (Spencer and Pahl, 2006:69), in telling about these rituals respondents were able to 'display' that their relationships fit the cultural ideal of friendship well. By indicating rituals that supported emotional sharing and support (share/support/vent rituals), they were able to 'display' that their friendship involved confiding and trust, confirming them as 'soul mate' friendships. Further, by indicating different types of symbols (nicknames, gifts, special times) respondents proved to the interviewer that the friendship was also characterised by a level of commitment.

Finch argues that through the telling of stories 'people attempt to connect their own experiences... to a more generalised pattern of social meaning' (2007:78). The 'pattern of social meaning' here could be seen as the norms and values associated with friendship. As Morgan (2011) argues, relationships should be seen to be influenced by cultural definitions. Rituals should be seen to constitute some types of 'friendship practices' through which the respondents actively 'do' friendship, and the telling of these practices to the interviewer was how they 'displayed' them (p. 207).

Why 'display' may not work

Whilst an element of 'display' was present through the use of physical symbols and through narratives told in the interview, there were more indications of 'doing' friendship, rather than 'displaying'. Many of respondents noted that they felt they did not enact rituals or show symbols for the benefit of an audience. Jordanne noted:

> I think [thinking about it] makes me really wrapped up in how I look to other people, rather than thinking about how you actually feel? Are you happy or sad? So it changes how you feel about the relationship. Coz you think, this is who I'm seen to be friends with, not this is who I feel closest to.

There are several reasons why the concept of 'display' may not be so transferable. Finch (2007) questions whether there are ever practices that involve 'doing family' but not 'displaying family' (p. 79). She concludes that these practices are so well understood within the framework of family that they do not need to be 'displayed'. In friendship, we could argue that when practices are so well understood in the frame of friendship, they do not need to be 'displayed'. Having behaviours that support emotional sharing (share/support/vent rituals), a favourite song (cultural artefact) or nickname for an ex-boyfriend (personalised code) were such commonplace and recognisable aspects of friendship that my respondents did not need to 'display' them to an audience.

Further, the concept of 'displaying family' was proposed by Finch as a tool for sociologists to analyse the changing family structure and fluidity of family life (2007:68). Heaphy (2011) argues that the politics of personal life are important when thinking about when the 'displaying' of relationships may take on more or less significance. In family life, for example, the image of 'the family' remains central and powerful. The role of 'the family' has political and economic implications; both Morgan (2011) and Finch (2007) note the legal, economic and social need to define 'family'. It is difficult to imagine the same being done for friendships despite policy emphasis in social work on informal caring. Although we argue here that the friendships described were influenced by cultural ideals, friendship is not institutionalised to the extent that family is.

In this context, 'display' becomes important as individuals strive to conform to the powerful image of a 'proper' family (Finch, 2007). There may be more pressure to prove that your family works, because the cessation of that relationship seems impossible. In comparison, as much as sociologists such as Smart et al. (2012) or Davies (2011) would highlight the negative aspects of friendship, they still assert that in contemporary society friendship is seen to be 'highly positive, desirable… and chosen' (Davies, 2011:72). The chosen aspect of friendship is important because it goes hand in hand with the assumption that it can also be terminated. If relationships can be viewed as expendable and they actually didn't work, individuals would feel less of a need to prove that they did, and more of an inclination to instead simply end the friendship.

Conclusion

This chapter investigated the functions of rituals and symbols in female 'soul mate' friendships to determine what purpose was served by the enactment of ritualised behaviour and acknowledgement of symbols in friendship. It set out to determine whether the concept of 'doing' (Morgan, 1996, 2011) and 'displaying' (Finch, 2007) could be comprehensively applied to friendship, and how rituals and symbols play a part in this (if any).

This study adds to the depth of analysis of ritual and symbol function by assessing the externality of ritual and symbol function. Whilst individual rituals and symbols are informed by the personal experiences of the respondents, rituals and symbols as phenomenon access cultural ideals about expected friendship behaviour. Utilising Morgan's concept of 'doing' helped to theorise this externality. Rituals and symbols should be seen to constitute 'friendship practices' which are informed by a wider cultural ideal of friendship; how respondents should behave and what is expected of them. They actively engaged with their role as 'friend' by 'doing' activities and behaviours that proved they are worthy of having that label, such as task/

favour rituals, share/support/vent rituals and/or showing an awareness that a cultural artefact (such as a favourite song) has a symbolic meaning.

'Displaying' friendship, on the other hand, was not a strong theme as respondents did not engage with the concept and at many points disagreed that these rituals and symbols were carried out for the benefit of an audience. Finch asserted that, 'display' is provided as something that sociologists should objectively place upon practices, but never as something individuals actively identify themselves as doing. Although Heaphy (2011) discusses the issue of reflexivity within 'display', it is reflexivity of the relationship, not reflexivity of whether 'display' is happening. This then in turn raises the question of who decides when and where practices get deigned with the label of 'display'. Concepts found in the sociology of family were transferred to the sociology of friendship to see if they remained comprehensible. Contemporary families are seen to be fluid and flexible. Weeks et al.'s study (2001) on families of choice suggest that friends can provide the support generally assigned to the family. In this study, when describing their 'soul mate' friends, many parallels were drawn between them and family members or romantic relationships:

RACHEL: 'We speak literally almost everyday... that's why I think she's like a boyfriend'
MICHELLE: 'I would describe it as love, as odd as it sounds but not that kind of love... like family love'
SCARLETT: 'We're more like family, more like cousins that get along'

These are important findings when we think about how we work with young people who may be separated from their families and their networks. Whilst family and friendships are not the same, the need to establish intimacy and maintain it through relationships is ever important for young women's well-being, as evidenced here.

Applying research findings to professional practice

We make several recommendations for social work with young women as a result of this study:

- It is important to be aware of relationships beyond the traditional family network commonly conceptualised with social work assessment and care support. This study illustrates the significance of social relationships beyond the family and their functions in providing support for expressions of intimacy, agency and identities.
- There are significant challenges in making friends when young people are experiencing conditions where their normal networks have been disrupted. It is important to explore these and facilitate existing or new friendships as much as possible and to introduce these discussions into care and support planning.

- Conceptualising friendships highlights the ways that friendship experience is shaped by minority status and inequalities. Young people need support to develop cross group friendships which promote cultural competence or dialogue between different social groups and reinforce their own identities through the life course.

References

Allan, G.A. (1979) *A Sociology of Friendship and Kinship*, London, George Allan and Unwin Ltd.

Baxter, L.A. (1987) Symbols of Relationship Identity in Relationship Cultures, *Journal of Social and Personal Relationships*, 4 (3), 261–280.

Bell, R., Buerkel-Rothfuss, N., Gore, K. (1987) Did You Bring the Yarmulke for the Cabbage Patch Kid? The Idiomatic Communication of Young Lovers, *Human Communication Research*, 14 (1), 47–67.

Bell, R.A., Healy, J.G. (1992) Idiomatic Communication and Interpersonal Solidarity in Friends' Relational Cultures, *Human Communication Research*, 18 (3), 307–335.

Best, S. (2012) *Understanding and Doing Successful Research; Data Collection and Analysis for the Social Sciences*, Essex, Pearson Education Limited.

Betcher, W. (1987) *Intimate Play: Creating Romance in Everyday Life*. New York, Viking Adult.

Bruess, C.J.S., Pearson, J.C. (1997) Interpersonal Rituals in Marriage and Adult Friendships, *Communication Monographs*, 64 (3), 25–46.

Bryman, A. (2008) *Social Research Methods*, Third Edition, Oxford, Oxford University Press.

Collins, R. (2005) *Interaction Ritual Chains*, Oxfordshire, Princeton University Press.

Crosby, G., Clark, A., Hayes, R., Jones, K., Lievesley, N. (2008) *The Financial Abuse of Older People A Review from the Literature*, Centre for Policy on Ageing. London, Help the Aged.

Davies, K. (2011) Friendship and Personal Life, in May, V. (ed.), *Sociology of Personal Life*, Basingstoke, Palgrave MacMillan.

Dermott, E., Seymour, J. (2011) *Displaying Families; A New Concept for the Sociology of Family Life*, Basingstoke, Palgrave Macmillan.

Durkheim, E. (1918) "Le « Contrat social » de Rousseau." © www.mediastic.info.

Finch, J. (2007) Displaying Families, *Sociology*, 41 (1), 65–81.

Galupo M.P., Bauerband, A., Gonzalez, K.A., Hagen, D.B., Hether, S.D., Krum, T.E. (2014) Transgender Friendship Experiences: Benefits and Barriers of Friendships across Gender Identity and Sexual Orientation, *Feminism & Psychology*, 24 (2) 193–215.

Giddens, A. (1991) *Modernity and Self-Identity; Self and Society in the Late Modern Age*, Stanford, CA, Stanford University Press.

Heaphy, B. (2011) Critical Relational Displays, in Dermott, E., and Seymour, J. (eds.), *Displaying Families; A New Concept for the Sociology of Family Life*, Basingstoke, Palgrave Macmillan.

Hook, M.K., Gerstein, L.H., Detterich, L., Gridley, B. (2003) How Close Are We? Measuring Intimacy and Examining Gender Differences, *Journal of Counselling and Development*, 81 (4), 462–472.

Landman, R. (2014) A Counterfeit Friendship: Mate Crime and People with Learning Disabilities, *The Journal of Adult Protection*, 16 (6), 355–366.

Miller, J., Glassner, B. (2011) The "Inside" and the "Outside": Finding Realities in Interviews, in Silverman, D., (ed.), *Qualitative Research*, Third Edition, London, Sage Publications.

Morgan, D. (1996) *Family Connections*, Cambridge, Polity Press.

Morgan, D. (2011) *Rethinking Family Practices*, Basingstoke, Palgrave-Macmillan.

Neal, J., Brown, C. (2016) 'We Are Always in Some Form of Contact': Friendships among Homeless Drug and Alcohol Users Living in Hostels, *Health and Social Care in the Community* 24 (5), 557–566.

Pahl, R. (2000) *On Friendship*, Cambridge, Polity Press.

Pearson, J.C., Child, J.T., Carmon, A.F. (2010) Rituals in Committed Romantic Relationships: The Creation and Validation of an Instrument, *Communication Studies*, 61 (4), 464–483.

Smart, C., Davies, K., Heaphy, B., Mason, J. (2012) Difficult Friendships and Ontological Insecurity, *The Sociological Review*, 60 (1), 91–109.

Spencer, L., Pahl, R. (2006) *Rethinking Friendship; Hidden Solidarities Today*, Oxfordshire, Princeton University Press.

Stevenson C. (2013) A Qualitative Exploration of Relations and Interactions between People who are Homeless and Use Drugs and Staff in Homeless Hostel Accommodation, *Journal of Substance Use*, 19 (1–2), 134–140.

Suter, E.A., Daas, K.L., Mason Bergen, K. (2008) Negotiating Lesbian Family Identities via Symbols and Rituals, *Journal of Family Issues*, 29 (1), 26–47.

Tannen, D. (1990) *You Just Don't Understand; Women and Men in Conversation*, New York, Harper Collins.

Weeks, J., Heaphy, B., Donovan, C. (2001) *Same Sex Intimacies; Families of Choice and Other Life Experiments*, London, Routledge.

5 Home and 'hood'

Middle-aged gay men's stories of homes and neighbourhoods

Paul Simpson

Introduction

The friendship-based 'families of choice' of gay and lesbian individuals (Weeks et al. 2001) commonly enacted in domestic spaces are as much part of gay culture as gay bars (Gorman-Murray 2008a). More recent literature covering gay experiences of the home has been recuperative of queer identities (see Gorman-Murray 2008a; Pilkey 2015). It describes the challenges queer home-making presents to heteronormativity (heterosexuality as the benchmark of sexuality). This body of work offers resources to think with but curiously has tended to overlook how *ageing* affects queer stories of homes and neighbourhoods and in ways that involve ambivalence, risk and insecurity. In this chapter, instead, I highlight a range of stories about homes, kinship and neighbourhoods told by middle-aged gay men that address some of the problems absent from accounts of queering of the home. To deepen the understanding of middle-aged gay men's accounts of home and 'hood', I extend theorising developed by sociologist Pierre Bourdieu. Famously, Bourdieu focused on how cultural, symbolic, social and economic processes combine to *constitute* and not just reflect social class. I also extend this thinking by highlighting at strategic points how differences of age intersect with differences class, ethnicity and relationship status. The 27 men who featured in my original study of growing older as a middle-aged gay man were aged between 39 and 61 and lived in Manchester. Britain's third largest city has a developed gay culture consisting of the highly visible and internationally marketed 'gay village'. Other not so well marketed aspects of Manchester's 'gay scene' include spaces for 'casual' sex (saunas and cruising grounds) various social/support groups and social media.

The overarching thesis of this chapter is that middle-aged gay men experience homes and neighbourhoods as empowering *and* ambivalent, if problematic, spaces in various ways. The first argument in support of my thinking is that the narrative 'resources' acquired through the ageing process, what I call 'ageing capital' (elaborated more below) and, in particular, through involvement in friendship family are commonly implicated in the *differentiation* of ageing gay selves and forms of relating. Historically, for gay men and lesbians, creating 'families of choice' (Weeks et al. 2001) as distinct from biolegal families of origin, has been politically necessary given widespread homophobia and rejection or partial tolerance by the latter. Moreover, later in life, gay men's kinship networks enable them to develop new political, emotional, moral and epistemic resources to contest (gay) ageism and indicate the gains that can come with gay ageing. (Commonly this process is understood as loss, particularly of physical capital or attractiveness.) Thinking of the gains of ageing helps contest the cautionary stereotype of the lonely old queen getting his just rewards for a lifetime of promiscuity lived outside of 'normal' kinship, i.e. biological family. As will be seen, friendship family is also a space that not only enables critical questioning of heteronormative notions of family, but can also legitimate the practice of (tentative) experiments in non-monogamy.

However, the second part of my argument is that ageing capital is not uniformly empowering. Indeed, middle-aged gay men spread stories that are implicated in reverse ageism where younger gay men are stereotyped as self-obsessed shallow and yet to fully develop as human beings. But there is also a sense in which ageing capital is overwhelmed or compromised by disadvantaged access to or exclusion from friendship family for lack of socio-economic resources combined with cultural reasons, i.e. connected with ageist homophobia. 'Failures' of ageing capital were manifest in men's responses to experiences of gay ageism online and of ageist homophobia in neighbourhoods, both of which can render the home and locality sites of risk for some men. As well as challenging notions of home as space of freedom, self-expression and safety, such thinking marks material and discursive constraints on men's ability to mobilise ageing capital.

To develop the above-mentioned points, 'ageing capital' requires further explanation. The concept represents an age-inflected form of cultural capital – internalised knowledge of society influenced by experiences of ageing, class, gender and sexuality – and social actors can use this knowledge in social life and to one's benefit. This process results in thought and practice that become ingrained (though are not beyond the power to change) and are expressed subconsciously through bodily action (Bourdieu 1984). Such a formulation allows that individuals deploy different kinds and combinations of resources across different contexts, which have their own rules of the game (Bourdieu and Wacquant 1992). Research subjects could deploy interrelated forms of capital: economic capital (financial resources), cultural capital (as just explained), symbolic capital (connected with status or reputation) and social capital (one's social networks). Together, these forms of capital help structure what Bourdieu terms 'habitus' – deeply habitual modes of thought and behaviour. In the study, habitus and its constituent capitals were visible in accounts of the fit/disjuncture between the midlife/older body and various 'homospaces'. For example, falling short of the approved, athletic, youthful 'look' risked marginalisation in the more commercial, sexualised gay village and saunas. The perceived loss of physical or sexual capital (Green 2008) encouraged men to invest more in domestically staged relationships, though these relationships were more appreciated as a gain of ageing rather than mere consolation for loss (Simpson 2014, 2015). Furthermore, ageing capital can refer to emotional strength, self-acceptance, knowledge of (age-appropriate) bodily display/performance and management of the rules of the game that make up various culture realms – queer or otherwise.

To contextualise the empirical discussion, I provide a brief review of the key themes in literature concerning gay kinship and uses of the home and neighbourhood and then explain the research design. In the concluding sections, I summarise the theoretical points of learning for practitioners and provide some recommendations for social work practice.

Gay ageing, relations and homemaking: the literature

Scholarship on LGB&T ageing usefully addresses forms of exclusion – socio-economic (Boxer 1997), socio-psychological (Quam and Whitford 1992) and the double invisibility of LGB&T individuals on grounds of age combined with sexual and/or gender difference. However, much of this practical, policy-oriented work lacks a sustained theoretical focus (Simpson 2015), for example, see Cruz (2003). It relies on a narrow, common sense notion of gay ageing as 'accelerated' in a youth-obsessed culture. Put simply, in gay culture, individuals are considered old before their time and thus excluded (Bennett and Thompson 1991; Cruz 2003; Hostetler 2004). Whilst this can certainly be keenly felt and is a dominant story in gay male culture, such obvious thinking can obscure that over time men develop emotional, political and epistemic resources to negotiate and challenge the stigma of gay ageing (Berger and Kelly 2002).

Moreover, the value of friendship families has been addressed by gay-identified scholars on both sides of the Atlantic. For instance, Weston (1991) has explored the kinship practices of mainly middle-class and 'out' lesbian and gay individuals in San Francisco. In Britain, Weeks et al. (2001) have examined how the (relative) freedom from regulation by the state and biological family has meant greater opportunities for lesbian and gay individuals to be involved in newer 'experiments' in intimacy and kinship. However, as seen below, the ability to participate in this form of kinship is not equally available; participation being affected by the economic and cultural dimensions of social class (Carrington 1999; Cronin and King 2010). Whilst both these pioneering studies referred to older participants, ageing sexuality was not their central focus.

In terms of defining the home, it has been argued that this is a multi-scalar concept that can refer to belonging to a nation, region, locality or spirituality (Fortier 2001). For present purposes, I focus on sociological accounts of home as a material site of emotional performances, intimacy and identity-production. As reflected in my discussion below, and depending on subjects' social positioning, homes represent different meanings to different individuals (Gorman-Murray 2008b), which involves pain and entrapment as much as pleasure and autonomy. Much of the literature then on gay/ queer homes deals with them as spaces of identity construction and expression through practices that reflect differences of gender and sexuality (Gorman-Murray 2008a; Pilkey 2015). Social and cultural changes over time, especially since the beginnings of tolerance in 1990s Britain, have brought about resignification of gay men and the home. If in the 1950s gay men were presumed to lead secretive, atomised lives considered the opposite of heterosexually coded homes (Cook 2014), contemporary home-makeover TV programmes stereotypically associate gay men with the home, especially as gentrifiers and experts in interior décor (Gorman-Murray 2006c; Pilkey 2013). It has been noted that such narrow definitions reinforce the idea that 'normal' gays (commonly presumed young or ageless) are affluent and predisposed to creative, feminised styles of self-expression (Gorman-Murray 2011).

Moreover, there has also been some productive queer and feminist-inspired geographical work exploring how gay men incorporate aspects of the gay scene into home life and décor (Gorman-Murray 2006c). Such accounts indicate further possibilities for disrupting the 'heternormalized' nature of the home by use of material objects whose meanings are constitutive of gay identity (Gorman-Murray 2006a, 2007, 2008a, 2008b). Some such work has drawn attention to how older gay men's generational homemaking practices can offer protection from heteronormativity and gay ageism (Gorman-Murray 2013) to proclaim the value of gay ageing (Pilkey 2015).

However, there is also a strand of scholarship that opens up the understanding of queer homes and experiences of the neighbourhood as more ambivalent and compromised, if not distinctly problematic, spaces. For instance, Johnston and Valentine (1995) have highlighted how lesbian homes can be subject to the heterosexual gaze, which encourages women to 'de-dyke' living areas to which relatives and non-habitants are invited. Localities and public spaces are also commonly read as predominantly heterosexual, sometimes requiring discretion by gay men (Simpson 2012). More recently, Cook (2014) has focused on homes as sites of self-expression *and* risk. On this account, (older) gay men's homemaking practices combine the conventional and the queer, indicating a need to fit in and, simultaneously, stand out. This latter view resonates with my analysis, though my recognition of the two important shifts (from biology and bars to friendship family) like that of Pilkey (2013) adds a specific *temporal* dimension often missing from academic and practitioner writing about gay men's stories of the home.

Research methods and sample

Study participants' accounts of ageing were generated through semi-structured interviews. The method produced narratives that recognised ageing as social process and that different meanings are created by differently positioned individuals (Maxwell 1996). A purposive sampling strategy, involving various recruitment methods, was designed to accommodate key dimensions of difference (rather than representativeness) and avoid a homogeneous sample of white, middle-class individuals generally open about their sexuality that (over-)populate studies of gay men (Friend 1991). To this end, project publicity (a matching leaflet/poster) were disseminated among: personal networks of peer-aged men known to me (though not close associates); gay social groups, including one for gay men aged 40 plus and one for black men; a gay sauna and sex aids shop; and various gay bars which, from personal use/fieldwork I knew were associated with differently aged clienteles. This strategy was designed to sample for differences of age (whether early or late midlife), class (culturally working-class men might gravitate towards bars rather than social groups), relationship status and patterns of use of local gay cultures (e.g. partnered men might prefer social groups to bars and saunas). The publicity framed midlife as *relatively* porous – 'forty-ish to sixty-ish'. This accommodated participants' different parameters concerning middle-age. The publicity also invited participation from men regardless of 'background', i.e. class and race (Table 5.1).

In terms of relationship status, study participants indicated a varied landscape of intimacy that encompassed being single, coupled, somewhere in between and involvement in friendship family. The 17 respondents (two-thirds of participants) who were single may have been easier to recruit given greater opportunities to be involved in the gay scene. Six of the coupled interviewees (nearly a quarter of participants) were involved in longer-term relationships that ranged from one year to 27 years. In terms of ethnicity, the sample was largely 'white British' – 23 respondents (88%) – but one respondent self-defined as 'mixed race', another as 'oriental' and another as 'Irish'. A social/support group for black gay men was contacted, but this largely comprised younger men. Problems of accessing non-white, middle-aged informants might also arise from a sense of exclusion from white-dominated gay scenes and prioritisation of ethnic identity over sexuality (Carrabine and Munro 2004).

Following Bourdieu (1984), social class was defined in terms of related socio-economic and cultural dimensions. This was used to allocate participants to class categories as below (Table 5.2).

The sample was evenly spread across two socio-economic classes, but reflects the predominance of culturally middle-class men (most reported having *become* so through education) who described a range of interests/capacities,

Table 5.1 Recruitment of participants

Source	Number/percentage
Social groups (gay men 40 plus, alternative to commercial scene, HIV-related)	16 (62%)
Mixed-age village bars	5 (19%)
Personal networks (of associates and participants)	5 (19%)

Table 5.2 Participants' social class

Socio-economic dimensions		Cultural dimensions	
Middle-class	Working-class	Middle-class	Working-class
12 (46%)	14 (54%)	21 (81%)	5 (19%)

suggesting knowledge/competencies that enable sampling across a spectrum of activities. Socio-economic class was based on descriptions of employment records/trajectories (current and/or main occupation). Estimates of income were derived from whether men were/not in paid employment, working part/full-time and their opportunities for career development. The cultural dimensions of class reflect the kinds of habitual knowledge participants spoke of that could enable them to participate (or not) in various cultural pursuits. A liking for pop music, pulp novels (stereotypically associated with working-class taste) or military history (associated with middle-class interests/knowledge) were explored to see whether these interests were read at a meta-level in terms of political understandings.

In terms of the ethics and politics of research, possibilities for emotional harm were minimised by disguising personal details to preserve anonymity. Interview accounts are affected by my positioning as a white, middle-aged, educated working-class gay man. I provided the motive for the study, devised the questions asked and interpreted the stories told. However, participants' challenges to assumptions within interview questions encouraged refinement and reframing of subsequent questions and alerted me to a broader range of responses to ageing. Transcripts were provided inviting participants to excise over-disclosure and a progress report invited commentary on interpretations of participants' accounts. Such a strategy was designed to minimise inequalities of power between researcher and researched in terms of 'representation, authority and voice' (Sherman Heyl 2001: 378).

Research findings

Gay homes as empowering: differentiating friendship family

The first major shift in men's relational practices involved a gradual move away from biological towards friendship family. The local gay scene includes village bars, saunas, social groups and gay websites as well as friendship family and relational 'experiments' (Weeks et al. 2001), including non-monogamous ones. In consequence, and constituting a major difference between gay male and heterosexual relationships, the former generally make the transition to domestically oriented kinship later in life, often around the forties (Berger 1992).

Just as significantly, two-thirds of the sample ($n = 18$), and regardless of class and ethnic difference, described the heterosexually identified family home as a site of risk (Weeks et al. 2001). Because heterosexual family tended to deny or misunderstand gay identity, just over half of informants ($n = 14$) spoke of a gradual diminution of bonds with their family of origin.

> My mum and dad don't really understand my life. I care for them and help financially, But, my partner is the one I rely on emotionally... more than anyone and not just because he knows me better but because we both understand what being gay is about... If I mention some homophobic incident, he knows how to respond.
>
> (Ben 50)

Like most other interviewees, who cared and offered practical help on occasions, Ben uses ageing capital when he speaks philosophically of increasing 'detachment' from the family of origin as if this was a natural and unremarkable life-event. Ben's account indicates support for the view that lesbian and gay people distinguish friendship family for its 'ethic of care', offering mutual support in the face of prejudice, from its less trustworthy biolegal variant associated with an 'ethic of obligation' (Weeks et al. 2001). For Ben, a small friendship family included a close friend as well as his co-habiting civil partner. Parental lack of understanding or unwillingness to understand gay lives were contrasted with the understanding and support from a partner and family of choice, which indicates that peer-aged gay kinship acts as a supportive 'community of understanding' able to hear the struggles, pain and joy that characterise lived experience (Plummer 1995: 134). It is worth noting that couple relationships and friendship families did not just provide consolation for the diminution of relations with the family of origin. As Ben suggests, peer-aged friendship families can help middle-aged gay men develop the emotional and political resources (a form of ageing capital) to challenge homophobia and claim validity for their kinship (Weeks et al. 2001). It is not surprising then that relationships with parents and relatives were typically described as limited to exchange of Christmas greetings and attending weddings and funerals.

The second major shift in gay midlife concerned a gradual move away from the gay village/bar scene:

> I don't go out on the scene a great deal these days. We've got different interests now. We like to have dinner parties (chuckles)... and we invite our lesbian friends over quite a bit... Actually, I like staying in on a Saturday night now. I've mainly grown out of the bar and club scene... I don't feel as though I'm missing out anymore... I just feel that age fades into the background here... I find that having people like this around makes me care less about how I'm seen in the village.
>
> (Jamie 54)

Similar to Ben's story of moving away from the family of origin, Jamie accepts the shift away from the gay bar scene towards the home calmly as a natural development of the gay ageing process (Berger 1992). The bar scene was something one might 'grow out of'. For Jamie, the spaces of friendship family are differentiated morally from the gay village scene because they are less age-conscious and thus freer from ageist scrutiny (Grossman et al., 2000). In the more convivial spaces of dinner parties with lesbian friends (a newer development for Jamie), age too is unremarkable and 'fades into the background' and enables Jamie to feel more confident (or less perturbed) about how he is viewed in the gay village. The transition from bar/nightclub scene to home here represents less withdrawal from social engagement with gay others than use of ageing capital creatively to recreate a gay scene that is now more focused on the home. As Ben's and Jamie's stories suggest, friendship family and homes (and those of significant others) can function as spaces for self-expression in ways that reference mutual understanding and support, sexual politics, intimacy and building self-esteem. As such, they are vital, sustaining sources of social, reputational and cultural capital.

Further, friendship family in a more hybrid form (combining friends and relatives) featured in Pete's account of caring for his 80-year-old father. This story provides a recognizably middle-class form of differentiation through use of ageing capital:

> I'd describe my network of friends as varied… a family of choice. One of my friends… has quite a few lesbian friends… And she wants us to set up a housing co-operative… involving, different generations… to provide a more supportive environment as you get older, which I would seriously think about in the future… And I've got two lesbian friends who will come and look after him if I need to get away for a few days. [Later during interview]…If he's feeling like it, I take my father out for a pub lunch if a friend comes round. Generally speaking, his needs come first… 'cause that's what he needs at his age. But, I'm also very clear about my own needs and try to ensure that these are met as far as I can… One thing I have learned from associating with my father and his friends is that there is a sense in which age is irrelevant… [Later]… There's much more to you than your body… There's your mind, personality, relationships… Overall, I give priority to my relationships.

Pete's story of investment in an eclectic friendship family includes his father (and some of his father's friends) from whom he has learned about ageing and valuing difference. Unlike many other study participants, an ethic of care and friendship are extended to a biological relative, which also involves mutual negotiation of personal needs. This account recalls Spencer and Pahl's (2006) take on contemporary friendships thought to consist of 'personal communities', not restricted to a particular form of affinity and characterised by people who represent different meanings to the person

concerned. Clearly, the gay home (or gay-friendly home in this case) provides a measure of security – enabling men to 'be themselves' without anxiety or need for self-surveillance (Gorman-Murray 2008a). The reference to
lesbian friends who provide informal though important respite care invokes
a sense of communitas often considered absent from the bar scene.

However, as a white, middle-class graduate, Pete's story suggests strate-
gising from a social position that combines a sense of self-value with a wish
for equality. Indeed, his narrative invokes a form of age-inflected, middle-
class cultural capital (e.g. the 'housing cooperative'). Three years prior to
interview, Pete, who could not afford early retirement, gave up a career in a
reasonably well-remunerated public service post to become a live-in carer.
This decision indicates a form of ageing capital that has involved Pete thinking through his own values and goals in midlife and in ways that avoid an
unwanted form of self-control. This was also evident in Pete's reference to
the importance of inner qualities of authenticity ('mind' and 'personality')
and his decision to prioritise relationships (more collective projects) over
more individualised, gay-approved body projects considered obligatory on
the youth-oriented gay scene (Simpson 2013; Slevin and Linneman 2009).

Ambivalences, exclusions and risk

The resources of ageing were also used in more ambivalent ways that were
discernible in tentative claims to differentiation from conventional forms
of intimacy by informants who were partnered but who practiced a form
of non-monogamy. Nevertheless, such accounts, expressed regardless of
class and race, challenge dominant thinking that sexual relations are only
legitimate when mutually exclusive and indicate possibilities for considering
non-monogamy as an alternative form of ethical relationship (Klesse 2007).
As Bill (55) exhorted: 'Don't do monogamy unless it is a genuine desire'.
Informants' age-inflected political and epistemic claims concerning sexual
ethics question the notion that non-monogamy *necessarily* entails an amoral
separation of sex and emotions (Anderson 2012). Indeed, Bill spoke of the
importance of being 'emotionally rather sexually faithful' to a partner,
which involved honesty about sexual experiences with others. Such accounts
represent claims concerning rights to sexual play with unknown/barely
known others without guilt or fear of being labelled 'superficial', calculating
or promiscuous:

> Y'know, you're playing these board games and somebody will signal to
> you and you'll go upstairs for a bit of hanky-panky. Me and me part-
> ner have had the odd threesome... He's not jealous at all... If he sees
> someone looking at me, he'll say, 'Go with him. Go on!' [Laughs]...
> I have had the odd one or two [sexual encounters] but I've not told him...
> He might have done. I'd rather not know, to be honest. And I'd rather he
> didn't know. What's the point?

It appears that the strength of Jamie's relationship and the interpersonal resources, involving mastery over sexual jealousy and the trust that he and his partner had developed, enabled both parties to enjoy this situation singly and as part of a 'threesome' with or without the partner's co-presence at the scene of the actual encounter. Whilst non-monogamy may represent an alternative form of sexual politics, it can also be regarded in gay male culture as an inauthentic relationship (Anderson 2012). Jamie's 'don't ask, don't tell' stance concerning opportune non-monogamy indicates how it functions in more cautious, problematic ways and, again, indicates limits on abilities to mobilise ageing capital.

Reflecting ambivalence around non-monogamy in a different way, Vince (49) explained, in light of his sexually-limiting complications of his HIV status, that:

> A relationship that's ideal for me at my age is one that is more than friends but less than lovers in a sexual way... I want somebody who is more constant in my life... a partnership. And even if, because of my health, we don't have sex, that's fine with me... I would certainly make allowances for him to see other people for sex if he's uncomfortable having it with me. But, if there was any emotional involvement, I wouldn't be happy with that.

Whilst Vince desires the constancy of partnership, he was prepared to forego sex with a partner and tolerate a partner having sex with unknown others. Although Vince strikes a forbearing note, acceptance of a partner's non-monogamy in return for physical affection and emotional fidelity is highly contingent. Willingness to 'make allowances' indicates that, in the absence of his health problems, monogamy would be the norm. Further, the relational arrangements envisaged would involve the imposition of constraint on any partner who would be required to avoid emotional entanglements and thus be required to turn any sexual partner(s) into mere instruments of pleasure, which might deny the feelings of both parties. The above-mentioned conspiracies of silence and pragmatic approaches to non-monogamy indicate further evidence of the fragile, contradictory character of interviewees' generational claims to self-value, knowledge of self and other and to authenticity in how they manage (courtesy of ageing capital) the relations that form gay culture.

Homes as sites of constraint and risk

Self-created friendship family is not equally available to all. Older gay people's capacities to mobilise the resources of ageing are contingent *and* 'uneven', reflecting socio-economic and cultural inequalities (Heaphy 2007) and indicating limits to the queering of homes (and neighbourhoods). Some men experienced significant restrictions on, if not exclusion from, friendship family. In line with Heaphy's theorising, such exclusions were largely attributable to cultural reasons connected with homophobia (Lewin 1998) and socio-economic ones (Carrington 1999) where being economically working-class could be exacerbated by relationship status as 'single'. In effect, these factors could combine to frustrate or even thwart men's capacities to mobilise the resources of ageing.

In contrast to Pete's narrative earlier about eclectic friendship family, Bill, a graduate who had been long-term unemployed because of health reasons, described separation from people with whom he had once been more closely socially involved:

> If I only had a nicer house and more money... The people I knew in this position tend to be more home-based... less scene-oriented... They tend to do more the dinner parties, barbecues, which I can't really do... They are owner-occupiers... house with garden... They're in and out of each other's houses a lot.

Effectively, Bill's long-term reliance on social security benefits and living in tower-block, social housing excluded him from reciprocation within middle-class, gay social networks – the affluent, coupled dinner party/barbecue circuit. He later described how his separation was exacerbated by his nominally single status, even though he was involved in several longer-term erotic friendships. His situation denied him access to social, economic, cultural and symbolic capital that might alleviate/compensate for material disadvantage. Indeed, Bill considered that his socio-economic situation and relationship status was responsible for prolonging his dependence on Manchester's 'gay village' bar scene.

In terms of cultural constraints, Alec, (46), who described himself as 'mixed race', spoke of the difficulties of negotiating a 'double life' that involved rigid separation between a coterie of peer-aged gay men who understood his sexual difference and heterosexual friends from his church and country of origin. The latter, nonetheless, provided a spiritual connection and freedom from racism, though lacking in gay culture (Fish 2008). Alec's double life was recounted as necessary given rejection by erstwhile friends from his cultural background. Such experiences could be marginalising and discouraged Alec from exercising a need for deeper participation in his church: 'I just turn up to mass then go home'.

In contrast to Gorman-Murray's (2006c, 2008a) (largely white, middle-class, Australian) interview samples, participants in my study spoke of homes and neighbourhoods in ways that suggested a greater plurality of experience. Indeed, the safety of the home was affected by experiences of the online gay scene. Although this scene offered opportunities for socio-sexual networking, study participants commonly spoke of it as a site of moral, relational, economic, reputational and sexual risk (see Mowlabocus 2010) as well as threatening intrusion into what they understood as private/personal space:

...sometimes all that people are looking for with online dating is people they can meet up with... Sometimes it's below 30 and in most cases it's definitely someone under 40.

(Alec)

I have blocked younger men who have played games with me. And I would certainly block anyone if they were after money.

(Marcus 47)

On Gaydar, it's just a cock... they very often don't provide a picture of the face.

(Jeff 48)

I probably mistrust people that would... want to have sex with me after such a short length of time... immediately. If you can make that decision so quickly, you can go off it again just as quickly... And you think, 'are they just, novelty seekers'?

(Chris 48)

The above criticisms indicate that the online gay scene is understood as the opposite of gay 'community' and obliges middle-aged/older gay men to negotiate various forms of risk (related to ageism and objectification) where individuals are reduced to their chronological age and/or body parts (Mowlabocus 2010). The virtual gay scene is characterised as constraining, discomforting, dehumanising and exclusionary on account of attempts by younger others to manipulate for personal gain and its capacity to render human relations emotionless and disposable (Klesse 2007). Alec's statement shows how middle-aged gay men are differentiated in a negative way and excluded from online sexual citizenship by younger men. Marcus' words suggest an age and class-tinged form of differentiation in the shape of anonymous, younger 'gold-diggers', which reinforces divisions between men of different generations. As announced in Jeff's comment, experiences of ageism on the virtual scene are largely attributable to over-reliance on the visual (Mowlabocus 2010) that focuses on the body/surface self and the superficial. This tyranny of the visual and objectification of body parts (commonly associated with younger men) could obscure appreciation of the more 'real', rounded (middle-aged) person. This kind of account, indicating ageing capital, implies a moral claim for a more holistic notion of the erotic beyond the fragmented, fetishised 'cock shot' or the demands of (younger) fickle, calculating sexual 'novelty seekers'. The above-mentioned narratives suggest that the home as space of emotional safety and autonomy is seriously compromised, even morally contaminated. They also draw attention to how middle-aged gay men's reliance on stereotypical ideas about younger gay men is implicated in ageism towards the latter, suggesting that gay ageism works multidirectionally (see also Simpson 2014).

Moreover, ageism towards middle-aged (or older) gay men could be combined with racism (Simpson 2014) and at times internalised by non-white gay men themselves. Whilst Alec spoke of enjoying gay social media, he declared:

> It tends to be mostly white but once in a while you get Asian, black and mixed-race people saying that they only want white men to be friends or date with... People can be more direct... less polite about this online.

Whilst the online gay scene had led to sexual adventure for Alec, contradictorily, it also figured in his account as a space where certain gay men are differentiated and rejected in a more overt fashion that dispenses with customary civility that applies in face-to-face interaction (Mowlabocus 2010).

Despite gains in self-worth, the security of the home and sense of belonging in the neighbourhood could be threatened by neighbours' age-tinged homophobia. Indeed, there is evidence that that homophobic intimidation is more likely to come from neighbours than strangers (Mason 2005). Alec's passion for photographing 'real life' situations on his housing estate resulted in accusations that he was photographing children 'for sinister purposes'. Interest in photographing the local area and its people was misconstrued as evidence of paedophilic intent, which suggests the continuation of a form of ageist homophobia that conflates ageing gayness with paedophilia, or the need to recruit to a gay cause and away from the natural heterosexual pathway. In turn, this led to threats to Alec's life and obliged him to take up residence on the other side of the city. Similarly, following an abortive police investigation instigated by the local Social Services Department of a consensual relationship with a man in his twenties with learning difficulties, Les (53) had felt obliged to leave his hometown to seek refuge in Manchester where he was unknown:

> I really did love the guy to bloody bits... We had penetrative sex... and I always consulted him first, every time... But, I was taken down to the police station and accused of male rape... He'd moved in with me... and I did this in consultation with Social Services... And I said, 'Look as long as I can have some support from you to help look after him...' I got nothing from them apart from alerting the police...

Social Services had been notified of Les' situation by the younger man's parents who were concerned that their son was being exploited. Les' story indicates the persistence of an ageist homophobia based on stereotypical assumptions about older gay men as predatory. Les reported having moved away from his hometown before any recriminations occurred. But homophobia (covert and overt) persists in more affluent areas. When considering buying home in a less familiar district to escape neighbours' homophobic intimidation in a middle-class area, Warren (52) and his peer-aged partner took the precaution of 'gaying' or outing themselves to their prospective new neighbours in order to sound out their reactions. It is significant that the couple felt obliged to resort to confessional tactics to establish the most basic security.

Implications for social work theory

Middle-aged and older gay men's stories of homes and neighbourhoods reflect the diversity of their social positioning and indicate the freedoms that men can forge, as well as the constraints, possibilities for exclusion and risks they can encounter. In terms of theoretical knowledge useful to practitioners, friendship family does important political and emotional work in empowering middle-aged gay men who generally felt unable to rely on their family of origin or younger gay men for support. Involvement in this kind of kinship does not merely compensate for the loss of physical capital on the gay scene, but indicates creative reconfiguration of men's gay scenes and social and cultural lives over time and their extension to domestic spaces. Such families enable men to express their 'authentic' selves, freed from the ageist scrutiny they encounter on a more youth-oriented gay commercial scene of bars, saunas and websites. Friendship family can also be characterised by an 'ethic of care' and mutual understanding (Weeks et al. 2001) rather than an 'ethic of obligation', which often applies to families of origin. This form of kinship also serves as critical space to develop the resources of ageing (Heaphy 2007) – the knowledge, emotional resources and political ideas needed to contest homophobia, gay ageism and to resist pressures towards monogamy.

However, the resources of ageing and ability to create friendship families are uneven and reflect dominant cultural and socio-economic inequalities that relate to differences and divisions of social class, exacerbated by homophobia. The forms of exclusion and risks identified represent constraints on middle-aged gay men's capacities to mobilise the resources of ageing. Simultaneously, they mark limits to the dominant idea of homes and neighbourhoods as spaces of self-expression and empowerment.

Applying research findings to professional practice

Practitioners supporting middle-aged and older gay service users should:

1   Recognise that middle-aged/older gay men are not a homogeneous group, but are differentiated by intersecting differences of class and race which influence who experiences isolation. Simultaneously, practitioners should be aware that men have developed emotional and other resources over time and previous experience of stigma in relation to sexuality can now be used/converted to counter the stigma of gay ageing. Approaches to support should be differentiated accordingly.

2   Develop strategies with service users to counter the stigma of gay ageing, both online and on isolation generally, though positive choices not too connected should also be respected.
3   Positively recognise and avoid subconscious judgement concerning involvement in non-monogamous relationships.
4   Inform and support men in claiming rights to financial support or other support in kind that might enable them to stay connected.

References

Anderson, E. (2012). *The Monogamy Gap: Men, Love, and the Reality of Cheating.* Oxford, Oxford University Press.

Bennett, K and Thompson, N. (1991) Accelerated Ageing and Male Homosexuality: Australian Evidence in a Continuing Debate, *The Journal of Homosexuality* 20(3–4), 65–75.

Berger, R. (1992) Research on Older Gay Men: What We Know; What We Need to Know, in Woodman, J. (Ed.) *Lesbian and Gay Lifestyles: A Guide for Counselling and Education,* New York: Irvington Publications Inc, pp. 217–234.

Berger, R. and Kelly, J. (2002) What Are Older Gay Men Like? An Impossible Question? *Journal of Gay & Lesbian Social Services,* 13(4), 55–64.

Bourdieu, P. (1984) *Distinction: A Social Critique of the Judgement of Taste.* London: Routledge.

Bourdieu, P. and Wacquant, L. (1992) *An Invitation to a Reflexive Sociology.* Chicago, IL: Chicago University Press.

Boxer, A. (1997) Gay, Lesbian and Bisexual Aging into the Twenty First Century: An Overview and Introduction, *International Journal of Sexuality and Gender Studies,* 2(3–4), 87–97.

Carrabine, J. and Munro, S. (2004) Lesbian and Gay Politics and Participation in New Labour's Britain, *Social Politics* 11(2), 312–327.

Carrington, C. (1999) *No Place Like Home: Relationships and Family Life among Lesbians and Gay Men.* Chicago, IL: Chicago University Press.

Cook, M. (2014) *Queer Domesticities: Homosexuality and Home Life in Twentieth Century London.* London/New York: Palgrave Macmillan.

Cronin, A. and King, A. (2010) Power, Inequality and Identification: Exploring Diversity and Intersectionality amongst Older LGB Adults, *Sociology* 44(5), 876–891.

Cruz, J. M. (2003) *A Sociological Analysis of Ageing: The Gay Male Perspective.* New York: Harrington Park Press/Howarth Press.

Fish, J. (2008). Navigating Queer Street: Researching the Intersections of Lesbian, Gay, Bisexual and Trans Identities in Health Research. *Sociological Research Online,* 13(1), 12.

Fortier, A.-M. (2001) Coming Home: Queer Migrations and Multiple Evocations of Home, *European Journal of Cultural Studies,* 4(4), 405–424.

Friend, R. (1991) Older Lesbian and Gay People: A Theory of Successful Aging, in Lee, J. (Ed.) *Gay Midlife and Maturity.* San Francisco (CA): Haworth Press, pp. 99–118.

Gorman-Murray, A. (2006a) Gay and Lesbian Couples at Home, *Home Cultures: The Journal of Architecture, Design and Domestic Space,* 3(2), 145–168.

Gorman-Murray, A. (2006c). 'Homeboys': Uses of Home by Gay Australian Men. *Social & Cultural Geography*, 7(1), 53–69.

Gorman-Murray, A. (2007) Contesting Domestic Ideals: Queering the Australian Home, *Australian Geographer* 38(2), 195–213.

Gorman-Murray, A. (2008a) Reconciling Self: Gay Men and Lesbians Using Domestic Materiality for Identity Management, *Social & Cultural Geography* 9(3), 283–301.

Gorman-Murray, A. (2008b) Masculinity and the Home: A Critical Review and Conceptual Framework, *Australian Geographer*, 39(3), 367–379.

Gorman-Murray, A. (2011). 'This Is Disco-wonderland!' Gender, Sexuality and the Limits of Gay Domesticity on 'The Block.' *Social & Cultural Geography*, 12(5), 435–453.

Gorman-Murray, A. (2013). Liminal Subjects, Marginal Spaces and Material Legacies: Older Gay Men, Home and Belonging, in Taylor, Y. and Addison, M. (Eds) *Queer Presences and Absences: Time, Future and History*. London: Palgrave Macmillan, pp. 93–117.

Green, A. (2008) The Social Organization of Desire: The Sexual Fields Approach *Sociological Theory*, 26(1), 25–50.

Grossman, A, D'Augelli, A., and Hershberger, S. (2000) The Social Support Networks of Lesbian, Gay and Bisexual Adults Aged 60 and Over, *Journal of Gerontology: Psychological Sciences,* 55B(3), 171–179.

Heaphy, B. (2007) Sexuality, Gender and Ageing: Resources and Social Change, *Current Sociology* 55(2), 193–210.

Hostetler, A. (2004) Old Gay and Alone: The Ecology of Well-Being among Middle-Aged and Older Single Gay Men, in De Vries, B. and Herdt, G. (Eds.) *Gay and Lesbian Aging and Research: Future Directions*. New York: Springer, pp. 143–176.

Johnston, L. and Valentine, G. (1995) *Wherever I Lay My Girlfriend, that's My Home*, in Bell, D. and Valentine, G. (Eds) *Mapping Desire: Geographies of Sexualities*, pp. 99–113.

Klesse, C. (2007) *The Spectre of Promiscuity: Gay Male and Bisexual Non-Monogamies and Polyamories*. Aldershot: Ashgate Publishing Ltd.

Lewin, E. (1998) *Recognizing Ourselves: Ceremonies of Lesbian and Gay Commitment*. New York: Columbia University Press.

Mason, G. (2005). Picture of Hate Crime: Racial and Homophobic Harassment in the United Kingdom. *Current Issues in Criminal Justice* 17(1), 79–95.

Maxwell, J. (1996) *Qualitative Research Design*. London: Sage Publications.

Mowlabocus, S. (2010) *'Gaydar' Culture: Gay Men, Technology and Embodiment in the Digital Age*. Farnham: Ashgate Publishing Ltd.

Pilkey, B. (2013) Queering Heteronormativity at Home: Older Gay Londoners and the Negotiation of Domestic Materiality. *Gender, Place & Culture: A Journal of Feminist Geography* 21(9), 1142–1157.

Pilkey, B. (2015). Reading the Queer Domestic Aesthetic Discourse: Tensions between Celebrated Stereotypes and Lived Realities. *Home Cultures*, 12(2), 213–239.

Plummer, K. (1995) *Telling Sexual Stories: Power Intimacy and Social Worlds*. London: Routledge.

Quam, J. and Whitford, C. (1992) Adaptation and Age-Related Expectations of Older Gay and Lesbian Adults, *The Gerontologist*, 32(3), 367–74.

Sherman Heyl, B. (2001) Ethnographic Interviewing, in Atkinson, P., Coffey, A., Delamont, S., Lofland, J., and Lofland, L. (Eds.) *Handbook of Ethnography*. London: Sage Publications, pp. 369–383.

Simpson, P. (2012) Perils, Precariousness and Pleasures: Middle-Aged Gay Men Negotiating Urban 'Heterospaces', *Sociological Research Online* 17(3), www.socresonline.org.uk/17/3/23.html.

Simpson, P. (2013) Alienation, Ambivalence, Agency: Middle-Aged Gay Men and Ageism in Manchester's Gay Village, *Sexualities* 16(3–4), 283–299.

Simpson, P. (2014) Differentiating Selves: Middle-Aged Gay Men in Manchester's Less Visible 'Homospaces', *British Journal of Sociology* 65(1), 150–169.

Simpson, P. (2015) *Middle-Aged Gay Men, Ageing and Ageism: Over the Rainbow?* Basingstoke: Palgrave Macmillan.

Slevin, K. and Linneman, T. (2009) Old Gay Men's Bodies and Masculinities, *Men and Masculinities* 12(4), 483–507.

Spencer, L. and Pahl, R. (2006) *Rethinking Friendship: Hidden Solidarities Today.* Princeton, NJ/Oxford: Princeton University Press.

Weeks, J., Heaphy, B. and Donovan, C. (2001) *Same Sex Intimacies: Families of Choice and Other Life Experiments.* London: Routledge.

Weston, K. (1991) *Families We Choose: Lesbians, Gays, Kinships.* New York: Columbia University Press.

6 Transgender people negotiating intimate relationships

Damien W. Riggs, Henry von Doussa and Jennifer Power

Introduction

Given the relationship between discrimination and poor mental health, it is perhaps understandable that much of the research to date focusing on transgender people has concentrated on the mental health of this population. Such research has been important for documenting experiences of marginalisation and victimisation, and for identifying the needs of transgender people in terms of mental health service provision (see Riggs, Ansara & Treharne, 2014, for a summary). Yet this focus on discrimination and mental health only speaks of one – albeit significant – aspect of the lives of transgender people. Much overlooked are the experiences that transgender people have of negotiating intimate relationships. To contribute to the growing body of research that has sought to correct this imbalance, this chapter begins by first providing an overview of previous literature on the topic of transgender people and intimate relationships, before reporting on findings from an Australian qualitative study focused on the topic. Importantly, the findings suggest both that understanding transgender people's experiences of intimacy cannot occur absent of an understanding of the effects of discrimination, but that recognising the impact of discrimination does not explain all there is to know about transgender people's experiences of intimacy. Beyond the impact of both discrimination and cisgenderism, for many transgender people experiences of intimacy are fulfilling and meaningful. The chapter concludes with recommendations derived from these findings for clinicians who work with transgender clients.

Introduction to previous research

Transgender people's experiences of intimacy as documented in previous research tend to be divided into four themes. The first theme emphasises the effects of cisgenderism upon transgender people in terms of intimacy. The second theme documents the effects of gender dysphoria upon some transgender people's capacity to negotiate intimate relationships.

The third theme highlights the impact of medical aspects of transition-ing upon some transgender people's experiences of intimacy. Finally, the fourth theme emphasises the unique and positive ways that many trans-gender people negotiate intimate relationships. These four themes are explored in turn.

Impact of cisgenderism upon intimacy

Cisgenderism is defined as the "the ideology that delegitimizes people's own understanding of their genders and bodies" (Riggs, Ansara & Treharne, 2014). Such delegitimisation takes a number of forms, and includes people referring to transgender people as not 'real' men or women, transgender bodies being treated as fetish objects and can include more generalised neg-ative or violent responses towards transgender people.

In terms of transgender people's experiences of intimacy, research by Tobin (2003) suggests that, in some cases, cisgender partners of transgender people contribute to the delegitimisation of their partner's gender identity. This occurs, for example, when a transgender man is treated as female or referred to as such in intimate encounters with a cisgender partner. This often occurs when anatomy typically viewed as female (i.e. a clitoris, vagina or breasts) is referred to as such by cisgender partners, despite many trans-gender men re-gendering these body parts as masculine (a topic explored in more detail in the fourth theme below).

In terms of the fetishisation of transgender people, research by Riggs, von Doussa and Power suggests that many transgender people find it difficult to negotiate intimate relationships with cisgender partners due to the percep-tion that their bodies are fetishised, which they see as a barrier to meaningful intimate relationships. Tompkins (2014) argues that, on the one hand, the treatment of transgender people as desirable solely on the basis of their trans-gender status is fetishising. On the other hand, Tompkins suggests that stat-ing that a transgender person's status is irrelevant denies the lived realities of transgender people and ignores the specificity of transgender embodiment and intimacy. In between these two polarised positions, Tompkins suggests, can lie a genuine attraction by some cisgender people to people of a diverse range of embodiments, in which such diversity is respected without being fetishised.

Finally, in terms of the impact of cisgenderism, Gamarel, Reisner, Lau-renceau, Nemoto and Operario (2014) suggest that negative societal attitudes towards transgender people impact upon transgender women's relationships with cisgender men. Specifically, they suggest that negative attitudes may be internalised by both transgender women and their partners, and that this can impact upon relationship satisfaction and mental health. As they sug-gest, a decrease in relationship satisfaction and reduced desire for intimacy can especially impact upon how transgender women view themselves and their bodies in terms of intimacy and self-esteem.

Effects of gender dysphoria upon intimacy

The language of 'dysphoria' in relation to transgender people is widely contested. Primarily, such contestation stems from the fact that the diagnosis of 'gender dysphoria' is seen as pathologising, and the requirement of diagnosis to access services is seen as marginalising. For many transgender people, however, a sense of dysphoria is keenly experienced and impacts upon willingness or capacity to enter into intimate relationships.

For example, Tobin (2003) suggests that some of his transgender participants were unwilling to enter into intimate relationships because of a sense of dissatisfaction or discomfort with their bodies. Importantly, some of his participants negotiated alternate ways of thinking about their bodies that allowed them to experience satisfaction in intimate encounters (a topic explored further in the final theme below). Nonetheless, for many of his participants, a sense of dysphoria reduced their capacity or willingness to even entertain the possibility of intimate encounters with other people.

An additional concern noted in previous research in terms of dysphoria, as documented by Doorduin and van Berlo (2014) in their research with transgender men, is that for many transgender people, feelings of dysphoria can also impact upon how intimacy is experienced. Doorduin and van Berlo suggest that some of their participants who had managed to negotiate intimate encounters with cisgender partners felt that during the experience they were not in control of their body and its responses to intimacy, and that this led to the encounter being akin to a rape. Importantly, as Doorduin and van Berlo note, "they felt not so much raped by their partners as raped by the *situation itself*" (original emphasis, p. 660). These findings demonstrate that for some people, the experience of dysphoria (which is arguably 'the situation' being referred to) has an extremely negative impact upon experiences of intimacy.

Effects of medical aspects of transitioning

For many transgender people, taking hormones and/or gender affirming surgeries are an important aspect of transitioning. Whilst this is not true for all transgender people, research documenting experiences of intimacy amongst transgender people has tended to include participants who have undertaken at least some aspects of medical transition. This research highlights two interrelated consequences of medical transition for expressions and experiences of intimacy: (1) changes to physical arousal and its impact upon sexual desire and sexual practices and (2) psychological and identity changes resulting from medical aspects of transitioning.

In terms of physiological changes, Doorduin and van Berlo (2014) report extensively on the differential effects of hormones upon transgender men and women. The latter, they suggest, often experience a decrease in sensitivity and arousal whilst the former experience greater sensitivity and desire for intimacy. For some of the transgender women in their sample, the reduced degree of arousal was desirable, as in the past they had found erections to be distressing, whilst other transgender women in their sample found reduced arousal to be distressing. Another point of difference was that orgasms for transgender women who had commenced hormones tended to last longer than they had in the past, whilst for transgender men orgasms were briefer though more intense.

Brown's (2010) research with cisgender female partners of transgender men indicates that some such women struggle to adapt to changes in their partner's arousal as they go through medical aspects of transition. Specifically, some of the women Brown interviewed reported that their partners became more demanding and less emotionally connected to them during sex, which impacted negatively upon their relationship. For some cisgender women, then, medical aspects of transitioning as undertaken by their transgender partners are viewed as a barrier to intimacy.

Finally, in terms of changes wrought by medical aspects of transitioning upon intimacy, Hines (2007) suggests that for many of the older transgender women she interviewed, their relationships with their wives changed following medical transition. Hines suggests that the quality of the relationship changed, though not necessarily for the worse. For many of her participants, whilst there was a reduction or cessation of physical intimacy (and especially sex), there was often an increase in tenderness and the strength of the caring relationship between her transgender participants and their wives.

Unique and positive negotiations of intimacy

Emerging within research on transgender people and intimacy is a clear and consistent narrative that many transgender people find creative ways to negotiate intimacy both prior to and following transition, and that for many transgender people this leads to positive and fulfilling experiences of intimacy.

A strong narrative across research focusing on transgender men is the importance of being perceived of and treated as a man by intimate partners. Research by Tobin (2003) and Schleifer (2006), for example, suggests that for some transgender men, comfort with receptive vaginal intercourse with cisgender men becomes viable if the transgender man feels that they are viewed and treated as a man by their intimate partner.

This relationship between bodily comfort and being correctly perceived leads some transgender men to re-gender particular body parts so as to facilitate perceptions of their bodies that align with their gender identity. So, for example, both Brown (2010) and Edelman and Zimman (2014) report that some transgender men refer to their clitoris as a dick or their breasts as their chest, and thus use language to refer to sex acts that relate to this terminology (so referring to oral sex performed on a transgender man as a 'blowjob'). This re-gendering of particular body parts serves an important role in making intimate encounters viable for transgender people who may not yet have commenced or may not plan to commence medical aspects of transitioning.

Finally, Bolin's (1988) research undertaken with transgender women suggests that for women who have not undertaken gender affirming surgeries, the penis can be re-gendered as a female organ, and thus remain a source of pleasure that is not psychologically distressing. For many of Bolin's participants, whilst vaginoplasty was seen as desirable, it was also seen as potentially unlikely (particularly with regard to the costs associated with it). Finding positive ways to view their penis was thus an important approach to making space for intimacy and sexual fulfilment in their lives.

Research project

The findings reported in the following section are derived from a research project undertaken by the authors, which focused on Australian transgender people's experiences of parenting, relationships with families of origin and intimate relationships. The project involved both an online survey (see Riggs, von Doussa & Power for findings from the survey) and a series of interviews undertaken by the second author. Ethics approval for the project was granted by the second and third authors' institution. With regard to the interviews, participants were primarily sourced via the online survey. Upon completion of the survey participants were asked to indicate if they were willing to be contacted for a follow up interview to explore in greater depth the topics addressed by the research project. In addition to those participants recruited via this method (10), a further two participants were recruited via snowball sampling from one of the initial participants, and an additional participant was recruited via a call for participants disseminated via an email network.

In total, 13 interviews were undertaken. These followed a semi-structured interview protocol. The focus of the analysis below is on responses to a particular series of interview questions related to intimate relationships. Participants were asked to describe their experiences of negotiating and being in intimate relationships, including both positive and negative experiences. The interviews were transcribed verbatim by a paid transcription service. The first author then read responses to these interview questions repeatedly to identify common themes across the interviews, keeping in mind the themes identified above from previous research. Five themes were identified through this process. Of these, two aligned to a certain degree with previous research, namely (1) Negative effects of cisgenderism (with specific regards to the fetishising of transgender bodies) and (2) Negotiations of intimacy across transitioning. Three additional themes were identified: (1) Pragmatic decisions about non-intimacy, (2) Normative expectations in the context of intimacy and (3) Intimacy between transgender partners. These five themes are now explored in turn, utilising selected representative extracts.

Findings

Negative effects of cisgenderism

Similar to previous research, participants who reported negative experiences of negotiating intimate relationships with cisgender partners emphasised how transgender people are at times treated as fetish objects. In the first extract below, Elizabeth notes that as she desires an accepting and honest relationship, she feels it is important to disclose her status as transgender. Doing so, however, means that she becomes vulnerable to people who would treat her as a fetish object, which means she is no longer seen as a person or a woman in their eyes:

> ELIZABETH: If I put myself on [an online dating site], they have only limited labels so you're identifying as transgender or transsexual or something like that. If I identify as that then you get typically some guy, quite often creepy guys that are interested in that as a fetish, as some sexual turn on thing and then I'm not a person or a woman anymore it's a real fetish thing. So it's a real conundrum because if I want to be open and honest, I want to get the person that I'm ultimately looking for, if I put on there as my real person they won't accept me for who I am, so it's just hard work it really is.

In the second extract below, Tom notes the same binary identified by Tompkins (2014), namely that if he actively names himself as a transgender gay man, then there is the possibility that his cisgender male partners may only be interested in him because he is transgender, rather than as a person (mirroring Elizabeth's concern above). On the other hand, not disclosing his transgender status would potentially deny the specificities of his embodiment as a transgender man:

> TOM: So when I did finally transition I did find it a lot more easier to make casual relationships I would say online, especially, because I found a lot more gay guys are just upfront about having a casual relationship. But I don't think that was so great for my self esteem because the way I was doing it was setting myself up as a novelty, as like a trans guy, so I'm different from other guys. I would have people who were interested in me just because I was trans rather than interested in me as a person. So again that wasn't particularly satisfying and for a long time I was mostly single.

These two extracts highlight the specific challenges that transgender people face when attempting to negotiate intimate relationships. Importantly, these challenges are the product of cisgenderism and the ways in which transgender bodies are delegitimised or seen in stereotyped ways. These extracts also highlight the double-edged sword of openness: both research and community advocates emphasise the importance of disclosure to potential cisgender partners so as to avoid negative responses (Belawski & Sojka, 2014). Yet the accounts provided by Elizabeth and Tom suggest that disclosure may not always lead to trans-positive acceptance: it may instead lead to fetishisation.

Negotiations of intimacy across transitioning

The extracts included in this theme again echo previous research in terms of highlighting the effects of hormones upon transgender people's experiences of intimacy. In the first extract, Sarah suggests that hormones render 'relationships post transition in technicolour', an evocative description of the power of hormones to change both a person's physicality and also their experience of their physicality:

> SARAH: Before I transitioned most of my emotions were like, suppressed, put behind a dam wall so to speak. I didn't want to deal with them, I couldn't deal with them. And after I transitioned that dam wall started to crack and break and emotions started pouring out. So my relationships became more intense and with the new hormones through my body my body became more sensitive so intimate relations so to speak were heightened a lot. So I would say that my relationships post transition like, in technicolour or high definition whereas before they were standard definition. It was just like, they were much more crisp and real.

Hamish, in the following extract, also emphasises hormones as producing a new form of 'intensity' in regards to embodiment, but also that transitioning meant that he had to adjust not just physically, but also psychologically to different ways of being in the world:

> HAMISH: So, what does transitioning mean for me now? Well it's an interesting journey. I think because I'm still earlier on in the journey, it continues to change and evolve, but I think when I first came out, I wasn't passing at the time and I didn't really get noticed a lot by gay men. That's very different now. So, it is, it's a huge adjustment to be honest. Look, it's an adjustment with the hormones, because the hormones are intense and it's been an adjustment in terms of my physicality and the cultural differences of coming from like a lesbian community to a gay male community is very different. It's highly sexualised; it's much more physical based.

An important recommendation often made to transgender people as they transition is to prepare themselves for the challenges that come with moving social groups. Whilst as critical scholars we might decry claims to essentialist gender differences, there is nonetheless a truth, as expressed by Hamish, in the *socialisation* of particular groups. In other words, without relying upon an essentialist notion of what it means to be 'male', we can acknowledge, along with Hamish, that the experience of moving from one particular social group ('lesbian community') to another ('gay community') brings with it differing demands in terms of negotiating intimate relationships.

Pragmatic decisions about non-intimacy

To a degree, the present theme echoes the findings of Hines (2007), in that her older female transgender participants reported that physical intimacy often declined or ceased between participants and their wives. Different in the present theme, however, is the arguably pragmatic decision by some of our, again older female, participants to eschew intimate relations, and to instead focus on other aspects of their lives that gave them meaning:

> STACEY: Something that came up in conversation today was the question of "What's your sex life like?" [On a community panel recently] three of us pretty much identified as asexual in that it's not a huge driver in our lives. We've had so many other issues to address that throwing that into the mix is so irrelevant. In terms of looking for another partner I've got no interest in that whatsoever. One of the other panel members has got no interest in that whatsoever. Each of us have had long term relationships that have ended for various reasons. In two of our cases we remain very good friends with our partners. One was same sex, mine was heterosexual and what we've decided anecdotally is that there's far less emphasis on sexual relationships of any description. We're far more interested in living full lives in terms of our professional lives, our friend networks than looking for sex and I think in the public's imagination the only reason we are like we are is because we're looking for some sort of compatible sex partner and I think that's a fallacy. That's a bit of mythology going on there. It's only anecdotal and we've compared notes on various circles of friends that each of us have it's very low on the agenda, incredibly low.

As Stacey notes, amongst her cohort of friends, the perception that transgender women all seek sexual partners is a fallacy. Instead, her emphasis is on other determinants of a 'good life'. Frances too, in the following extract, emphasises the importance of focusing on the good already in her life, though to a degree her shift away from a focus on intimate relationships leaves her nonetheless feeling lonely:

> FRANCES: I'm actually quite lonely. I would have to just perhaps admit you know, I'm quite lonely and I have always been lonely because I have never had, you know, a nice relationship since [I was with my

child's] mum and we were really loving you know... It's a small demographic you know, it's a narrow demographic you know, of like
transwoman interested in lesbian woman or other transwomen. And
you know, maybe if I tried harder, I don't try very hard, you know,
like, I'm on this social networking site and if I pay money, which I'm
too stingy to pay the money... There's a number of women that are
saying they would like to meet me, I don't know. I don't know why
I don't do it. It might be $70 really well spent, who knows. But look,
we're off to [an event] on Thursday, my son and I and although you
know, I haven't had an intimate friendship through the people I've
met at [the event previously], I have met really nice people my age who
I really like. And look, that's okay, that's kind of just about enough
for me I think. You know, you can't have everything?... I've got a lot
now and it's sort of like, I just - there's something about not expecting
everything. That sort of, I think it's the way I think. It's like, you're
doing pretty well Frances, you've got a lot of good things happening
and good friendships you know. Do I need to get into some strange
fucking, you know, needy kind of relationship with a person whose
needs sort of overtake my own and those of my - relationship with my
son. You know, disrupt this calm, you know, and this established lifestyle? You know, my painting is like my girlfriend. You know, I'm with
her all the time, always thinking about her. I'm always mixing colours
in my mind, you know. You know, I'm not really - it's not making me
very sad really but sometimes I've just got a bit of a hole there.

The account provided by Frances exemplifies our use of the word 'pragmatic'. Whilst some participants like Stacey above provided no clarifiers
to the choice of celibacy, other participants like Frances emphasised that
whilst technically they had chosen celibacy, they did so in order to avoid
heartbreak, or being treated as a fetish object, being rejected by potential
partners, or just avoiding the complications and demands that can come
with an intimate relationship. This is clear in the emphasis by Frances upon
feeling lonely, despite all that she has in her life. To a degree, then, whilst we
respect the decisions made by participants such as Stacey and Frances, we
also raise the question as to the degree to which some decisions are made in
a context of cisgenderism and where older transgender women in particular may struggle to negotiate accepting and affirming intimate relationships
(Riggs & Kentlyn, 2014).

Normative expectations in the context of intimacy

The extracts identified as part of this theme all centre upon normative expectations placed upon men's and women's bodies, both by participants and
by their intimate partners (or a combination of both). Such expectations became especially problematic for some participants when their desires didn't

necessarily accord with what is normatively expected of their bodies. In other words, normative expectations associated with bodies read as female and bodies read as male conflicted with the desires of some participants to be treated as, or to be able to engage intimately as, men or women. In the first extract below, Janet emphasises that her desire to be a sexually dominant woman seeking intimacy with men means that she encounters particular 'types' of men who don't accord with what she is seeking:

> JANET: I like my sex drive and I like having sex, but I don't like getting fucked up the arse, I'm a bit of a top so I kind of sexually am a little bit limited with guys. I either find two lots of guys: I find guys that just want me to fuck them up the arse and my idea of a man isn't someone taking up the arse, I mean no problem with that, it's kind of fun, but I want my man to be a man if I'm going to be the woman. What else, then I'd either get the guy who wants to fuck me hard and I don't like it up the arse so of course that wasn't going to do it for me either. Then everyone goes well, why don't you go and get [gender affirming surgery] like most of my friends went and did and I'm like I don't think that's kind of working either.

Perhaps particularly important in this extract is the injunction that Janet experiences from her friends, namely to 'solve' the problem she faces in meeting appropriate men by having gender affirming surgery. This type of injunction to surgery reduces Janet's desire to a particular normative form of embodiment required of women who desire men, rather than encouraging alternate ways of thinking about intimate relationships between men and women, and how they may be configured sexually. Hamish too, in the following extract, highlights how normative expectations placed upon him by people who read him as female had previously limited his relationships with men:

> HAMISH: I identified I guess probably as a straight girl up until about 19, at which point I realised that my sexuality wasn't as clear cut as that. And I think probably looking back in retrospect, that's when some of this stuff actually started to come up, but I just didn't have names for it. And what I knew was at the time that I would have relationships with men who sexually were compatible, all that stuff worked, but what didn't work was the energy around it and I'm a driven and ambitious kind of person and I felt very stymied by the role that I was expected to play as a woman in those relationships. It didn't work for me and it didn't work in my relationships with men and so I just think in my early 20s I was quite confused about what that meant and who I was and like I said, I didn't have a language, I didn't know trans men existed for a very long time.

Perhaps different to Janet's account of the expectations of others, the account provided by Hamish emphasises the utility of speaking with other

transgender people, which allowed Hamish to understand his identification
as transgender, and from there to be able to explore relationships with other
men in which he was recognised and treated as a man (as outlined in the previous extract from Hamish). Different altogether from Janet and Hamish,
however, is Zoe's account below, which emphasises her own normative expectations of how she should be treated by a male partner:

> ZOE: Whenever I think about – like at this point in time, where I am –
> relationships, I guess the thing, for me, would be that – I guess this
> is probably sexist on my own part. I have this image that came to
> me one day. I woke up with it so strong in my mind. Is that having
> my hair quite long in a ponytail, and it's over to one side and stand-
> ing at the kitchen sink doing dishes, and man coming up and put-
> ting his arms just around my waist. That's just what I want. That's
> just what came to me. That image, that daydream, whatever it was,
> made me happy. I guess that's what my fantasy would be.

To a certain degree, understanding and validating the accounts of some
transgender women runs counter to what we might understand as a feminist
account of gender relations. To a degree, we might, in general, argue for a
non-normative account of relationships between men and women: one that
doesn't reinforce gender stereotypes (and this was certainly the case in regard to Janet's account). At the same time, however, it is vitally important to
acknowledge that for some transgender women (and men), a normative experience of gender relations is what is desired, and perhaps indeed needed.
The account provided by Zoe thus challenges the normative imposition of
non-normative understandings of gender relationships between men and
women upon transgender people, and instead encourages a revisiting of the
role of gender norms in the lives of some transgender people.

Intimacy between transgender partners

This final theme speaks to the positive and supportive relationships that
some transgender people enter into with another transgender person. In the
one extract included in this theme, Tom speaks about the positives of being
in a relationship with another transgender man, but importantly, he also
acknowledges the differences between transgender people.

> TOM: [What is good about my relationship with my partner is that] he is
> another trans guy. Like we have that understanding and with other
> people, people can get it really well. Like they can understand being
> trans but I suppose there is always that sort of barrier where they
> don't fully appreciate what it means or what you go through and
> just having someone there for that support and has helped both of
> us I think. Also I think he's helped me reconcile being trans a lot
> more because whereas before I was not really meeting any other

trans people or really having much contact with them at all and it was like living a double life. I would go off to work when no-one knew I was trans and I would come home and I would just be by myself and that sort of thing and it was just sort of like as secret from my life or just something from my past. Whereas now I feel like I can be a lot more open about being trans and I've met a lot more other trans people as well.

As noted above, this extract is important because it highlights both the strengths of intimate relationships between transgender people, but also reminds us that the 'transgender community' is heterogeneous: it is comprised of people of varying experiences, interests and desires, and that two transgender people in a relationship does not mean that there will not be significant differences in terms of experiences. Nonetheless, as Tom's account demonstrates, intimate relationships between transgender people can foster a sense of being understood, of self-acceptance and of feeling connected to a broader community.

Conclusion

The findings presented in this chapter make a significant contribution to the developing focus on intimacy within the field of transgender studies. As suggested at the beginning of this chapter, a focus on intimacy (amongst other topics) is important, so as to provide a rich and holistic account of transgender people's lives, rather than solely focusing on mental health outcomes and their relationship to discrimination. Nonetheless, the findings presented in this chapter indicate that for the large part, transgender people's experiences of intimacy – particularly in relation to partnerships with cisgender people – must be located within the broader context of cisgenderism and the specific forms of discrimination that transgender people encounter. Whilst it is vitally important that the intimacies that transgender people diversely negotiate and experience are celebrated, it is also important to remember that such intimacies, even at their most positive, are often implicitly framed by gender norms and normative expectations of gendered embodiment.

In terms of clinical responses to the findings presented in this chapter – a focus for us as researchers and clinicians in the fields of public and mental health – there are many take home messages. The first has already been stated above, namely that understanding intimacies as experienced by transgender people must involve an awareness of the effects of cisgenderism: how it shapes individual's understandings of their bodies, how it constrains available ways of understanding and how it marginalises transgender people. At the same time, the findings indicate ways that clinicians can work with transgender clients to develop alternate ways of understanding their own bodies. Of course, many transgender people already do this, and discuss with their peers ways of re-gendering particular body parts. But as some of the interviewees indicated, not all transgender people are connected into transgender communities, and those who are may sometimes receive normative responses (such as the injunction to undertake gender affirming surgery). Knowledgeable and informed clinicians thus have a role to play in sharing information about alternate ways of thinking and talking about bodies.

In terms of the responses that transgender people receive from potential intimate cisgender partners, the findings presented in this chapter suggest that caution is warranted in regard to clinicians automatically assuming that the disclosure of transgender status will be productive. Whilst clinicians may presume that disclosure is a key way to ensure the safety of transgender people negotiating intimate encounters, this may not always be the case. Instead, it would appear important for clinicians to engage with transgender clients to weigh up multiple, potentially competing, factors when deciding whether or not to disclose. These may include potential risks to physical or psychological safety, the mode of meeting (online or in real life), previous discussions undertaken with potential partners (which may indicate attitudes held by them) and risk management plans (such as taking a friend along or meeting in a public place). Importantly, our suggestion here is not that transgender people should necessarily always be on guard when it comes to disclosing their transgender identity. In an ideal world, this should never be necessary. It is to suggest, however, that caution may be warranted in advocating for disclosure in all cases.

Echoing previous research, the findings also emphasise the importance of ensuring that transgender clients who are commencing hormone therapy understand the possible side effects, especially with regard to intimacy. Whilst generalisations must be undertaken with caution, research findings appear to indicate a relatively stable set of changes that occur for transgender men and women in terms of sensitivity in the genital region, desire for intimacy and experiences of intimacy. Without adequate preparation, these types of changes may be alarming and distressing for some transgender people. Discussing fully these possible changes is thus an important part of an informed consent model of transgender health care.

Conversely, it is also important to acknowledge that some transgender people may adopt a celibate or asexual identity upon transitioning. Indeed, of the survey conducted as part of this research project, 6.3% (10/160) of the sample identified as asexual (Riggs, von Doussa & Power). This should not be taken as indicating that transitioning was ill advised. Rather, it indicates that, as with any major life change, priorities will likely be re-evaluated, and the (often pragmatic) decision to focus on other things that give life meaning is valid and should be supported. This does not mean that, over time, some transgender people who for a period are asexual or celibate may not decide upon another path. Rather, it acknowledges that for those people who do adopt celibacy or asexuality, this requires support and understanding rather than the imposition of normative understandings of what constitutes 'appropriate' expressions of sexuality (Chasin, 2015).

Applying research findings to professional practice

* Those who work with transgender clients (including transgender clinicians themselves) must be mindful of the importance of engaging with transgender people's experiences of intimacy.
* Importantly, clinicians who undertake formal assessments of transgender people to support hormones and/or gender affirming surgery potentially already do this as part of a broader psychosocial assessment. The topic of intimacy in such assessments, however, is potentially developmentally normative and focused on evidence of dysphoria. In a sense, this focus is not inherently positive, and may indeed contribute to a negative perception of intimacy amongst some transgender people.
* Clinicians are behooved to also incorporate a positive focus on intimacy when working with transgender clients, so as to support such clients into the future to live fulfilling and meaningful intimate lives as they determine them to be.

References

Belawski, S.E., & Sojka, C.J. (2014). Intimate relationships. In L. Erickson-Schroth (Ed.), *Trans bodies, trans selves: A resource for the transgender community*. New York, Oxford University Press.

Bolin, A. (1988). *In search of Eve: Transsexual rites of passage*. London, Bergin & Garvey.

Brown, N.R. (2010). The sexual relationships of sexual-minority women partnered with trans men: A qualitative study. *Archives of Sexual Behavior, 39*(2), 561–572.

Chasin, C.J. (2015). Making sense in and of the asexual community: Navigating relationships and identities in a context of resistance. *Journal of Community & Applied Social Psychology 25*, 167–180.

Doorduin, T., & van Berlo, W. (2014). Trans people's experience of sexuality in the Netherlands: A pilot study. *Journal of homosexuality, 61*(5), 654–672.

Edelman, E.A., & Zimman, L. (2014). Boycunts and bonus holes: Trans men's bodies, neoliberalism, and the sexual productivity of genitals. *Journal of homosexuality, 61*(5), 673–690.

Gamarel, K.E., Reisner, S.L., Laurenceau, J.P., Nemoto, T., & Operario, D. (2014). Gender minority stress, mental health, and relationship quality: A dyadic investigation of transgender women and their cisgender male partners. *Journal of Family Psychology, 28*(4), 437.

Hines, S. (2007). *Transforming gender: Transgender practices of identity, intimacy and care*. Bristol, Policy Press.

Riggs, D.W., Ansara, Y.G., & Treharne, G.J. (2014). An evidence-based model for understanding transgender mental health in Australia. *Australian Psychologist, 50*, 32–39

Riggs, D.W., & Kentlyn, S. (2014). Transgender women, parenting, and experiences of ageing. In M. Gibson (Ed.) *Queering maternity and motherhood: Narrative and theoretical perspective.* Toronto, Demeter Press.

Schleifer, D. (2006) Make me feel mighty real: Gay female-to-male transgenderists negotiating sex, gender, and sexuality. *Sexualities, 9*(1), 57–75.

Tobin, H.J. (2003). Sexuality in transsexual and transgender individuals. Honors Thesis, Oberlin College.

Tompkins, A.B. (2014). "There's no chasing involved": Cis/trans relationships, "Tranny Chasers," and the future of a sex-positive trans politics. *Journal of Homosexuality, 61*(5), 766–780.

7 'Out' and about at work

Institutionalised heteronormativity on relationships and employment

Alfonso Pezzella

Introduction

This chapter will explore key concepts of LGBT employees and their experience of disclosing their sexual identity and/or orientation in the workplace. I present issues faced by LGBT employees in the workplace in relation to discrimination and bullying, relationships with colleagues and managers and the perceived impact of 'coming out' on their careers and succession planning. This focus on the issue of disclosure of LGBT employees about their sexual identify and/or sexual orientation to colleagues or managers and the barriers and benefits of disclosing one's sexual identity and/or sexual orientation, I argue, is important to mental health, social inclusion and well-being. The chapter will draw from available literature on the topic and on a case study of LGBT staff in a university from recent research conducted by the author.

Diversity management in the workplace has been the focus of many successful organisations by giving attention to addressing issues as a result of the evidence on workplace inequalities and disadvantages (Kelly and Dobbin, 1999). These have addressed areas such as gender, ethnicity, disability and age equality. However, less has been done to address the employment and workplace issues of sexual minorities, such as Lesbian, Gay, Bisexual and Trans* populations (LGBT). Over the past decade, there has been an increased interest in LGBT issues in social work research, education and practice. Despite change to legislations to protect LGBT rights and local policies within workplaces (such as, the Marriage (Same-Sex Couples) Act 2013; the equality Act 2010; Civil Partnership Act 2005; Gender Recognition Act 2004; Employment Equality (Sexual Orientation) Regulations 2003; Sex Discrimination (Gender Reassignment) Regulations 1999) research suggests that LGBT individuals are still victim of discrimination and bullying in the workplace, which has an impact on their general work-life balance and mental health: for example, in gendered patterns of hierarchy, occupational segregation, the predominance of heterosexuality, harassment and discrimination and in the questioning of work-life balance (particularly in relation to family responsibilities). These are, in turn, defined by and instrumental in reproducing social relations of age, class, disability, culture and ethnicity (Hafford-Letchfield, 2011). Despite the research findings on increasing acceptance of LGBT individuals, as well as the efforts of legal and mental health advocates to fight for equal rights of sexual minorities in the workplace, the choice to disclose one's sexual identity or not in the workplace remains challenging (American Psychological Association, 2009); causing gay and lesbian workers to question the 'risks' to their professional careers in disclosing their sexual orientation to the colleagues (Brewster, Velez, De-Blaere and Moradi, 2012; Chrobot-Mason, Button and DiClementi, 2002). In spite of the above description of the gains in legislation and rights to promote sexuality within particular areas such as employment, which have gone some way to transforming the everyday lives and experiences of lesbian, gay and bisexual people (Cocker and Hafford-Letchfield 2010), the choice to disclose one's sexual identity in every social role, whether in their personal life, social life or in the workplace, is still controversial (Barrett, Lewis, and Dwyer 2011; Gates and Mitchell, 2013; Gonsiorek and Rudolph, 1991; Jordan and Deluty, 1998; Morris, Waldo, and Rothblum, 2001; Schmitt and Kurdek, 1985). This may force gay and lesbian workers to weigh up the risk of 'coming out' to their colleagues, given the potential for this to affect their professional career and prospects.

Despite our progression in society in relation to LGBT rights and responsibilities and the level of education, promotion and awareness of the same, many of the younger generations are still uncomfortable with or unsure about homosexuality (Sharpe, 2002). This uncertainty of the non-heterosexual orientation usually results in discrimination and oppression. Apart from homophobia, which is the hostile reactions to lesbians and gays as expressions of irrational fear (Herek, 1984), factors such as religious and/or political beliefs and one's morals also reinforce these attitudes towards the LGBT group.

Background

Discrimination in the workplace

Lesbian, gay and bisexual employees are more likely to be a target of discrimination (American Psychological Association Task Force, 2009). The economic aspect of discrimination can include job loss or limitations in job promotion (Brewster et al., 2012). LGBT employees who disclose their sexual orientation are at risk of experiencing discrimination in the form of verbal attacks or physical threats (Gordon and Meyer, 2008). The negative attitude towards sexual minorities in the workplace has a negative impact on an individual's productivity, overall career development (Rostosky and Riggle, 2002) and general work satisfaction (Harbeck, 1997). However, if the workplace climate is tolerant and positive, the decision to come out can contribute to effective support networks, loyalty and higher job and life satisfaction (Brewster et al., 2012; Rostosky and Riggle, 2002).

Also, the concealment of sexual orientation is likely to decrease job satisfaction (Smith, Wright, Reilly and Esposito, 2008). On the one hand, the decision to disclose one's sexual orientation can be perceived by LGBT individuals as the only way to survive in the corporate world (Driscoll, Kelley and Fassinger, 1996). Those individuals who have decided not to disclose their sexuality are more likely to suffer from discrimination in the workplace. People have different reactions to the work environment according to their individual perception of existing or potential discrimination (Chung, 2001). Hence, management of sexual identity in the workplace is a complex phenomenon which includes more factors than just a decision to 'come out' or not.

Workplace climate, actual tolerance and levels of empathy towards colleagues have an influence on the mental health of LGBT individuals: stress levels, self-acceptance, quality of life and work satisfaction in general (Brewster et al., 2012). Homophobic attitudes raise potential threats to members of sexual minorities in terms of work related limitations: difficulties in peer and supervisory relationships, boundaries in promotion, job mobility and social benefits (Driscoll et al., 1996). According to one study, only 38% of LGBT workers feel free to disclose their sexual identity (Huebner, Rebchook, and Kegeles, 2004). Huebner et al. (2004) reported that 37% of men who took part in their research were victims of verbal and physical harassment. They also reported that younger men were more likely to report discrimination and were also more willing to disclose their sexual identity or orientation to colleagues in the workplace. LGB individuals often face bullying and feel unable to be open about their sexual orientation with colleagues and managers; 19% of LGB employees have experienced verbal bullying from colleagues, students or service users because of their sexual orientation in the last five years; 13% of LGB employees would not feel confident reporting homophobic bullying in their workplace and 26% of LGB workers are not at all open to colleagues about their sexual orientation (Stonewall, 2013, 2014, 2017).

In the United Kingdom, employers are slowing beginning to address LGBT sexualities and needs by making progress in managing workplace diversity. Many workplaces strive to achieve national recognition as 'diversity champions' and top the Stonewall 'Workplace Equality Index', an annual guide to the UK's top 100 'gay-friendly' employers. Stonewall, formed in 1989, is the largest LGBT rights organisation in the UK and in Europe, taking its name after the Stonewall riots in New York City (1969). Nevertheless, the 'gay-friendly' labels and awards do not guarantee a weakening or eradication of heteronormativity within the workplace (Rumens and Kerfoot, 2009), neither does it prevent any form of discrimination or phobias towards LGBT individuals. Some studies have revealed how gay-friendly organisations continue to discriminate against LGBT people (Giuffre, Dellinger, and Williams, 2008).

Equality recruitment and monitoring of diversity enables employers to examine the make-up of their workforce. Most organisations already collect demographic data of their employees, such as ethnicity, age, gender and disability. The Employment Equality (Sexual Orientation) Regulations 2003 do not, however, oblige employers to monitor the sexual orientation of staff and many do not. Having said that, monitoring sexual orientation can help an organisation identify, tackle and prevent discrimination against LGBT staff, which can affect job performance and productivity (Stonewall, 2006). Despite not having a legal obligation to monitor sexual orientation of their staff, employers must tackle sexual orientation discrimination in order to comply with the law and prevent discrimination. Nonetheless, this is sometimes difficult due to the lack of systems in place to prevent and address discrimination.

It is crucial for organisations to identify sexual orientation discrimination through monitoring, and tackling it, in order to build a reputation for valuing diversity and protecting its staff. Moreover, LGBT employees who feel their employer has an inclusive culture feel able to be themselves at work. Staff who are able to be themselves are happier at work (Stonewall, 2006).

Historically, homosexuality was considered a mental disorder until 1973 when the American Psychological Association (APA), along with other professional organisations (American Psychological Association, 2005; American Psychiatric Association, 1973; American Psychoanalytic Association, 1991, 1992; Conger, 1975; National Association of Social Workers [NASW], 2003), removed homosexuality from the Diagnostic and Statistical Manual of Mental Disorders (DSM) and the social movement against sexual discrimination began (Carr and Pezzella, 2017). Research has shown that discriminatory attitude of the society towards the LGBT population is still very prevalent as they are targets of considerable prejudice, which is manifested in a wide range of behaviours, from verbal expressions of dislike to violent attacks motivated by their sexuality or gender identity (Huebner et al., 2004; Subhrajit, 2014). It is crucial for organisations to support LGBT employees. Research suggests that LGB people are 50% more likely to develop long-term mental health problems, LG people are twice as likely (while bisexual people are four times as likely) to attempt suicide as people who identify as heterosexual. Additionally, 88% of trans* people have experienced depression compared to one in four of the wider population. More than 60% of trans* people have attempted suicide, and there is double the risk of drug and alcohol dependency in LGBT (Stonewall, 2015).

Impact of discrimination on the individual's psychological health and well-being

Mental health and well-being of sexual minority members is an under-research subject in the UK and other countries. Meta-analysis of studies on perceived discrimination and health (Pascoe and Richman, 2009) showed that discrimination has a negative influence on one's mental and physical health; in particular, heterosexism has a positive correlation with depression and psychological distress (King and Cortina, 2010). The decision of some LGBT employees not to come out and to pretend to be heterosexual is psychologically demanding and limits one's gender performance (McDermott, 2006).

The minority stress model by Meyer (2003) describes the impact of stigmatisation on LGBT employees' experience of discrimination stress. According to this theory, the psychological distress increases if individuals experience discrimination, hide or conceal their sexual identity and internalise negative social views on LGBT community. Members of sexual minorities use different types of coping mechanisms to deal with the stress of discrimination and one coping mechanism is positive reframing where a person learns from a negative experience and turns it into something positive. Positive outcomes correlate with reduced depressive symptoms and amelioration of stresses. Self-reinforcement disrupts negative stereotypes and transforms institutionalised stigmatisation into increased compassion to self and others (Meyer, 2003; Riggle, Whitman, Olson, Rostosky and Strong, 2008). However, some individuals avoid dealing with the psychological influence of experiences of rejection (Riggle et al., 2008).

In the context of higher educational institutions (HEIs) openness of LGBT staff can have positive and negative impacts on their psychological well-being due to specific features of the work environment. However, the openness of LGBT educators makes them a role model for both heterosexual and homosexual students, but the decision to come out is not always welcomed by all students. Additionally, LGBT educators can face the problem of the management of the professional boundary between themselves and students.

Coming out

Sexual identity is a complex biological and social characteristic, which influences the individual's choice of emotional and/or physical attractiveness. Sexual identity influences sexual orientation of the person, which can be heterosexual, homosexual, bisexual or questioning. The term questioning sexual orientation is used for individuals who are not compelled yet to call themselves homo- or bisexuals and unsure about their sexual identification (Martin and Murdock, 2007). Historically, gender identity referred to two main gender identities, male and female. However, gender identity is not a set as one might think, in fact, there are at least 71 gender categories in which people identify themselves. For example, cisgender, queer, intersex, asexual, pansexual, trans and so on.

'Trans' or 'trans*' with an asterisk can be used as shorthand to reflect the full spectrum but is not exclusive to: transgender, transfeminine, transmaculine, transsexual, transvestite, genderqueer, genderfluid, non-binary, genderfuck, genderless, agender, non-gendered, third gender, two-spirit, bigender, androgynous and gender non-conforming. In summary, transgender activists acknowledge the complexity of the area and the difficulties in negotiating through a vast range of terms (Beemyn, 2003, 2005; Beemyn and Rankin, 2011; Butler, 1988; Feinberg, 1999; Hafford-Letchfield, Pezzella, Cole and Manning, 2017; Valentine, 2007;). Trans* people experience similar challenges to LGB people; however, their needs might be different and need different approaches. For example, a person who wishes to transition from male to female will need practical support, such as time off work in order to achieve this. Furthermore, they might need reasonable adjustments to their work programme or environment to meet their needs in their current gender. This is a key issue for employers to address and specific policies or protocols are required to address these specific trans* needs in the workplace. Moreover, there is still an abundance of prejudice, ignorance and stigma towards trans* people, and often their needs are difficult to understand, leading to transphobia. In this chapter, you will notice that the acronym LGBT has been referred to LGB and T, taking the T out of the LGBT umbrella term because often T's needs have been neglected and policies and/ or laws do not necessary represent the T to address the full complexity and needs (Hafford-Letchfield et al., 2017).

To describe the process of acceptance and disclosure of one's sexual identity, the term 'coming out' is used. 'Coming out' in the workplace has a complicated structure for LGBT individuals, which influences different areas of their social life (Rostosky and Riggle, 2002), as well as psychological well-being and self-acceptance (Kertzner, Meyer, Frost and Stirratt, 2009). Institutionalised heterosexism and homophobia, along with self-doubt and lack of support, can stop individuals from disclosing their sexual identity to others in the workplace (Driscoll et al., 1996). Internalised homophobia can be developed by individuals in a heterosexist workplace that devalues and offends non-heterosexuals. It can be described as negative emotions and self-hate towards one's own sexual identification, which indicates psychological distress and lower self-esteem (Rostovsky and Riggle, 2002). Self-acceptance is one of the key factors in an individual's decision to disclose their sexual identity or not, along with rejection and reprimand (Driscoll et al., 1996).

The disclosure of sexual identity and orientation or 'coming out' has been identified as a key feature of the lives of LGBT individuals. When encountering new people, LGBT individuals need to make rational choices whether or not to disclose their sexual identity and/or sexual orientation, based on social roles and environment, gender, cultural and religious beliefs. One of the challenges within this is deciding whether or not to disclose one's sexual identity and sexual orientation in the workplace. Disclosure may, for example, increase the likelihood of a lesbian, gay male, or bisexual (LGB) worker to experience discrimination (Croteau and Lark, 1995; Croteau and von Destinon, 1994), job loss (Badgett, Donnolley, and Kibe, 1992; Bradford, Ryan, and Rothblum, 1994), verbal attacks (Bradford et al., 1994) or physical threats (Herek, 1995). Whilst the majority of evidence suggests a negative impact, there are some studies that report disclosure at work enhancing worker satisfaction, productivity and loyalty (Friskopp and Silverstein, 1995; Powers and Ellis, 1995).

Barriers to coming out

According to the research report of Equality Challenge Unit (2009), more than 89% of LGBT employees of HEI disclosed their sexual orientation to some colleagues and only 31% are 'out' to most people in their workplace. However, early-career workers rarely make decisions to come out compared to those who worked longer at HEI (Equality Challenge Unit, 2009).

Three main barriers to coming out can be named:

- The first concern is about employment security. LGBT employees on fixed-term contracts and early-career staff on probation assume that coming out can negatively influence their chance to get permanent, ex- tended or renewed contracts.
- Second, LGBT educators raise concern regarding their ability to fulfil teaching responsibilities when students might respond in a homophobic way in both formal and informal contexts.
- The third barrier for LGBT employees in HEIs refers to research in- terests in the areas where community can be circumspect about the re- searcher's sexual identity (for example, theology and religious studies).

Hence, because of the specific features of the work environment in HEIs, LGBT members can face additional barriers and discrimination factors which influence their decision on coming out. Coming out is a personal choice LGBT individuals are faced with. Coming out can result either in a very pleasant experience which can improve their relationship with col- leagues, or it could have the opposite effect and they could experience dis- crimination in relation to their sexual identity or sexuality. The process of disclosure is not always a positive one and, even being protected by diversity policies, LGBT educators have reported discrimination towards them, such as unpleasant assignments and negative gossip (Harbeck, 1997; Smith et al., 2008).

Positive impact on coming out

LGBT researchers usually pay little attention to positive aspects of LGBT employees' life. There has been little research into LGBT staff working in higher education and disclosing their sexual identity to colleagues (Equality Challenge Unit, 2009).

A national study of LGBT Educators' perception of their workplace climate (Smith et al., 2008) showed that teachers rated their work satisfac- tion higher if they considered themselves more 'out' in workplace. LGBT educators felt more comfortable being acknowledged for their successes when they disclosed their sexual identity to administrators (Harbeck, 1997). Members of sexual minorities find positive aspects of being a lesbian or a gay man in the domain of social support systems: belonging to a community and creating connections and families of choice. The process of 'coming out' involves personal changes and insights. Some respondents in the study of Riggle et al. (2008) reported the increase of self-awareness, compassion for others and empathy. As participants reported, authenticity and honesty are the most common feelings accompanied the process of one's disclosure. The changes in societal definitions of roles gives those who disclosed their sexual identity the freedom to express themselves emotionally, to explore their intimate relationships and, consequently, influence positively on the individual's well-being (Riggle et al., 2008).

LGBT stigma in the workplace

One of the causes of discrimination is social stigmatisation that applies to sexual minorities or non-heterosexual behaviour in general. Stigmatisation and/or labelling can be a stress factor for the whole group at both the societal level and at the individual level (APA Task Force, 2009). Heterosexism is a structural social stigma based on the belief that heterosexuality is the only right sexual orientation (Herek, 2007). It can be expressed in negative interpersonal interactions, by withdrawing of the LGB or T person from the social group (Rostosky and Riggle, 2002) or by employment of violence (Rostosky and Riggle, 2002), which can be described as enacted stigma (Herek, 2007). Social stigma can be adopted by the member of stigmatised group and developed into self-stigma when a person experiences negative attitudes towards oneself and/or members of the same minority group (Herek, Gillis and Cogan, 2009). However, the stigma competence model by David and Knight (2009) proposed that the mental health of LGBT people can be improved through positive change reduction of internalised stigma through acceptance of one's own sexual identity (APA Task Force, 2009). Apart from the individual factors, a strong feeling of social identity can have a positive influence on minority stress when community resources are used to respond to social stigma. Since the late 90s, mental health organisations are focused on offering help to sexual minorities to cope with social and internalised stigma.

Impact on promotion, risk of job loss and wages

LGBT individuals are at more risk of job loss than heterosexual colleagues: they have substantially lower salaries than heterosexual colleagues (King and Cortina, 2010). Twenty-three% of trans staff and around 4% of LGB employees were denied a promotion due to their sexual orientation and report discretionary pay raises. To take a closer look at the levels of negative treatment of LGBT staff in HEIs, take, for example, the rate of systematic institutional and implicit discrimination that was experienced by colleagues (33%), students (18%) and others (25%) (Equality Challenge Unit, 2009).

Some research demonstrates a difference in levels of salaries and renumeration between LGBT employees and their heterosexual counterparts. According to Elmslie and Tebaldi (2007), heterosexual men earn 23% more than homosexual men with the same level of education. However, wage discrepancies for lesbian employees are not that clear, as it can be explained by lower rates of participation in male-dominated fields and career interruption with maternity leave as a result of gender discrimination (King and Cortina, 2010). Moreover, some research shows that those who are closeted in their workplace have higher levels of job satisfaction than LGBT members who disclosed their sexual orientation (Ellis and Riggle, 1996; Lyons, Brenner and Fassinger, 2005) due to higher rates of pay and better job prospects shared with their heterosexual counterparts.

Covert discrimination of LGBT staff in HEIs has an impact on professional development of educators because of exclusion from social events that consequently becomes an obstacle for development of work-related and research networks. Due to the fact that informal exclusion is a form of discrimination which is not so obviously visible, proving it can be challenging. Fear of prejudicial treatment keeps employees from disclosing their sexual identity (Pitts, Smith, Mitchell, and Patel, 2006; Ragins, Singh, and Cornwell 2007). Many LGBT employees continue to face discrimination and exclusion as a result of heterosexism, cultural bias and religion-based discrimination (Giuffre et al., 2008). It is crucial for employers to be aware of this. One of the strategies used may allow space for informal LGBT societies or forums to take place in order to be more visible and support LGBT employees.

Work satisfaction and partnered relationship

Three factors contribute to work satisfaction: occupational environment and collegial acceptance along with personal needs. A study on lesbian identity and disclosure in the workplace (Driscoll et al., 1996) showed the significance of being able to express ones partnered relationships (an interpersonal, intimate relationship between two individuals who are not necessarily married or cohabiting) in the decision to disclose. For example, the longer one is in an intimate partnership, the higher the possibility that individual will disclose their identity in the workplace. Also, being in a partnered relationship was shown to correlate with occupational stress, e.g. the longer the individual is in a relationship, the lower the stress level (Driscoll et al., 1996). The interdependent nature of the partnered relationship has a positive influence on the disclosure decision making process, which helps to cope with work-related stress and to increase general work satisfaction (Rostosky and Riggle, 2002).

LGBT employees in HEIs

So far, the chapter has looked at LGBT issues in the workplace and the process of disclosing their sexual identity and/or orientation. The remainder of this chapter draws on some of my own research based in a university in the South East of England which explored (Pezzella, 2016) the barriers and benefits of coming out in the workplace, looking at HEIs and its impact on mental health.

The university environment might be seen as a place where there is freedom and respectful exchange of ideas (Iconis, 2010), as well as acceptance of individuals from different backgrounds. Unfortunately, this is not always the case. In fact, evidence suggests negative attitudes towards this group in both university and college campuses (Brown et al., 2004; D'Augelli, 1989a, 1989b; Iconis, 2010). The difficulties faced by the LGBT community in educational environments, such as universities, has become prevalent in recent years and is the main focus of research in this field (Arndt and De Bruin, 2006). One of the first studies in the field found that 26% of the LGB students in a university had reported cases of threats and verbal assaults (D'Augelli, 1989). Similarly, a survey by the same author, D'Augelli (1992), found that 77% of the respondents experienced verbal abuse and 27% were threatened with violence.

Juul and Repa's (1993) research suggests that educators who are out to students and colleagues have a higher job satisfaction and engage in the social and interpersonal role of being an educator. This study, however, did not address the climate factors that influenced the reasons for or against coming out and corresponding comfort levels.

A case study

Study design

The study adopted a mix-method approach comprising of an anonymous online survey and a further follow up in-depth interview. In the first study, all staff working at a HEI received an invitation to complete an anonymous online survey, and if they identified themselves as LGBT, they were asked to take part in the study. A general email was sent rather than targeting individuals or groups to minimise bias. After completing the online survey asking about demographic data and some qualitative questions, participants had the option to take part in the second stage of the research, which would involve a face-to-face interview. A purposive sample was self-selected from the wider university staff.

The university had approximately 2,000 employees, and taking into account that at least 10% of the population identifies as LGBT, the target population for this study was approximately 200 respondents. However, of those, the total number of participants that completed the online survey was 40. Of these, 22 identified as male and female (12 male and 10 female). Of those 22, eight left their contact details to be interviewed in the next stage of the study. Ten participants chose not to leave their contacts details but explained why. Comments were left, such as, 'I don't want to come forward otherwise I will be labelled as gay', or 'I am not out to my family and I don't wish to come out to colleagues'.

Ethical considerations

The project was granted ethical approval from the Social Work Sub Ethics Committee. The survey was mainly used to access LGBT individuals in the workplace, however, the researchers were fully aware of the possible consequences that completing a survey would have for LGBT individuals, such as being exposed to colleagues or labelled as either gay, lesbian, bisexual and so on, or being victim of discrimination. In fact, the researchers asked at the beginning of the survey why people did not want to take part in the research (those who did not) and one of the survey questions was about leaving their contact details and if they did not wish to leave their details, why they chose not to. Functions within SurveyMonkey were used to ensure that the IP was not tracked to ensure anonymity.

Despite all the precautions taken to preserve anonymity, the survey had a low response rate, suggesting there were still employees not wishing to disclose their sexual identity or sexuality in the workplace. Reasons might be different and/or personal, but interviews from the same study indicated a fear of being discriminated against or being labelled. Snowball technique was used in the second phase of the study, using participants who left their contact details. The snowball technique is often used in the studies recruiting LGBT people because participants are hard to find due to their 'invisibility' (Browne, 2005). Seventeen participants in total were recruited for the interviews, and of those, fifteen decided to take part in the interviews: eight female and seven male between the age of 24 and 54. In addition to the snowball technique, the researcher decided to come out, identifying himself as part of the LGBT community. This was crucial for building a relationship of trust with participants who told me that initially they were not sure about taking part in the research, but then they felt at ease in doing so knowing that the researcher was 'like them'.

The interviews were semi-structured, digitally recorded and lasted approximately 30–40 minutes. They encouraged participants to discuss the experience of their current and past working conditions and environment in relation to their sexuality. They also offered an opportunity to discuss their sense of self and professionalism, and discuss their mental health and well-being at work in relation to their sexual identity. Furthermore, with the literature review on partnered relationships in mind, specific questions were asked, for example, how many years they were in a relationship and how this influenced their 'coming out' experience. They were also asked if they had a supportive home environment in relation to their sexuality and whether this had an effect on their decision to come out or not at work. Finally, participants were asked how disclosing or not disclosing their sexual identify had either a positive or negative effect on their mental health and well-being.

Analysis

The interview transcripts were imported in NVivo 10 and they were then coded using thematic analysis (Braun and Clarke, 2006). The two researchers met on different occasions to discuss the project as it was developing and to ensure reliability of the findings.

Findings

Although most of the participants who took part in the interview stage were out in the current workplace, some had been out in their previous employment, therefore, during the transition to the new workplace it was easier to be out, and some decided to come out in their current employment. Six themes emerged from the data from both the survey data and interview data, however we will present only three major themes related to this chapter. Other themes were around students' support and coming out to students.

- Barriers encountered to coming out at work
- Fear of discrimination
- Perceived heterosexism
- Lack of understanding about bisexuality
- Fear of stereotyping
- Fear of religion-oriented bullying
- Office gossip, promotion potential
- Fear of students' reactions

Benefits to coming out at work

On the positive side, people who were out and open about their sexuality and sexual orientation reported what they felt were the benefits of this:

- Feeling able to be who you are was a reoccurring theme for all participants.
- Talking to colleagues freely about their personal life/partner.
- Not having to hide their personal life which would lead to 'enjoying social gatherings'.

Moreover, the study found that those who were not out and perceived as heterosexual by colleagues would often be victim of indirect homophobia, or witness 'straight talk'. One participant reported 'colleagues in the office think I am straight, so they are constantly talking about girlfriends and making comments on those gay boys who can't get a bird'. A participant explained 'I heard two female colleagues talking to each other, and they were talking about masculinity and one of them said "there are now real men around here" and they both started to laugh'. Thus, it is vital for employers to embrace diversity in full and have clear policies in place to support LGBT employees and minimise discrimination and bullying.

Theme 1: Inoculation

One of the main themes from the data was the sense of stability expressed by participants, a state where they felt like, in their experience of being gay, being discriminated against reached a point where 'they don't care anymore' about telling people or what people think. I have interpreted this as a form of inoculation. Inoculation is used in medical terms whereby a subject is given small amount of the virus so that the immune system gets used to it and produces enough antibodies. I use the term inoculation as it seems that participants built a form of resilience that they are now inoculated to 'being stigmatised' and they are fine with it. In fact, participants reported that all their life they fought for their place in society and they had experienced stigma and some form of homophobic talks that led them to not care anymore. In the words of some of the participants:

> I don't care what other people think about me anymore... This is who I am.
>
> (Gerry – Gay man)

> Pretty much a foregone conclusion...in school...anybody assume that I was gay anyway, so, there wasn't really a process of coming out.

Theme 2: Role model, peer and student support

Participants reported that one of the benefits of being out is the fact that they were able to support other LGBT colleagues who were thinking of coming out or having problems. They were able to provide moral support and act as a role model for both colleagues and students. A simple thing like wearing an LGBT badge or lanyard facilitates more visibility of the LGBT community.

> ...I think they definitely need role models... I think if there isn't a LGBT society I would be quite a disappointment...some people need that, they need to join it and they need to have support.
>
> (Laura – lesbian woman)

...in my social work career, LGBT students came to who were LGBT, because they felt it was important that students knew that, you know, members of staff were gay and it was a bit of "help" for them to know who to go and have someone to talk, for support of interests... but I haven't done that here yet...

(Silvia – lesbian woman)

Theme 3: Employer support

Another reoccurring theme was the help participants felt that they received from their employers. Most participants were aware of legislation on discrimination or homophobia/transphobia, however, the majority of them reported that they were not aware of any local policies or practical translation into support for LGBT staff who had experienced discrimination or bullying in relation to their sexual identity or sexual orientation.

...my sexuality I don't feel that it has impacted my work that much. I guess more on a personal level like a teamwork level where you watch the things you say or might hold things back...

(Nick – gay man)

Some academic staff did not feel supported in coming out to students as they felt their colleagues would not approve or feel that is was a breach of personal boundaries or unnecessary disclosure:

A lot of academic writers, this is a tradition in the social work in sort of [a] psychodynamic idea of you bring yourself as a blank sheet...don't give anything of yourself, really.

(Sue – lesbian woman)

Discussion

The above case study (Pezzella, 2016) suggests that despite policies and 'gay friendly' environments, people still do not feel at ease coming out in HEIs. This is due to the lack of knowledge and stigma towards LGBT, by colleagues and students. Stigma can manifest in many forms and can come from colleagues as well as students, particularly in institutions with different nationalities and cultural and religious backgrounds. Based on the study, I suggest that role models are also needed. Senior managers, for example, could be role models and be proactive in championing LGBT awareness to create a less hostile environment for LGBT employees. They need to be aware if any discrimination is happening; LGBT individuals might not feel confident in challenging or reporting this behaviour to a senior manager or Human Resources (HR), therefore managers must make it clear that they take homophobia seriously. Simple awareness workshops and teaching material for staff and students could prevent bias and challenge personal beliefs and stereotypes. Challenging homophobia and heteronormativity in the workplace is also very important.

Conclusions

It is clear from the issues addressed in this chapter that not all organisations pay enough attention to the sexual identity and orientation of their staff and associated issues with it. As seen in the case study in a HEI, homophobia, biphobia and transphobia remain a part of everyday culture in some workplaces. This is a neglected issue which requires urgent attention to ensure that LGBT rights in employment are recognised and promoted. Despite achievements in diversity, LGBT remains the last bastion of equality for employees and students alike in university education. Over a third of LGBT staff in HEIs is not aware of the existence of written policies on sexual orientation discrimination in their institution (Pezzella, 2016). The literature review on the experiences of LGBT workers shows a gap in knowledge of the experiences of staff working in higher education in disclosing their sexual identity to colleagues. Future research in this field can add to the effort to investigate the effects of the decision to come out in the workplace. The exploration of the experiences of sexual minority staff would enable organisations to provide a more effective specialist support structure and equality provision. Moreover, further research will also be beneficial to the organisations in terms of staff and student retention, successful communication of the information on equality policy, legal compliance and institutional reputation.

As mentioned above, LGB and T individuals are constantly making rational decisions on whether or not come out to family, friends and colleagues. As seen, this can be affected by many factors, including internalised homophobia, religion, culture, job satisfaction, promotion prospects and social relationships with colleagues in the workplace. Therefore, it is vital for social work practice and education to join hands and provide both educational material and policies to protect LGBT rights. Supporting colleagues, valuing their expertise and experience and role modelling LGBT inclusiveness are all key factors that we can portray in everyday life and in the work environment. Challenging discriminative behaviour as discussed previously, such as homophobic talks or indirect discrimination (such as 'there are no real men here') is everyone's business, not just in the interest of LGBT people. It is often a complex process to challenge personal beliefs and stereotypes, but as social care professionals, these beliefs need to be set aside when the interest and the priority is our service user. Whether it is a gay couple who wish to adopt, or a lesbian woman who finds herself homeless and kicked out of her family house because of her sexuality, social workers must be unbiased and support the person in need.

Stigma towards LGBT cannot be eradicated overnight and shifting cultural beliefs is a slow process that requires imaginative and creative methods to get students or the community involved to learn about LGBT individuals. Exposure to LGBT, through awareness workshops and campaigns, could facilitate this process.

Key recommendations for applying research to professional practice

* The implications for employment practice in social work
* Being aware as a social work student or educator of the rights of LGBT colleagues when we are working in higher education and ensuring that we enable and respect diversity of those leading as well as consuming education
* Thinking about the curriculum in Higher Education and Practice and the potential for the LGBT community developing these to show leadership and positive role modelling.
* Transferring the concept of coming out at work in different areas of the sector in social work and social care and learning from the case study.

Acknowledgements

The author would like to thank Professor Carmel Clancy at Middlesex University for her valuable guidance and support on the 'coming out in the workplace' project.

References

American Psychological Association. (2009). *Report of the Task Force on Appropriate Therapeutic Responses to Sexual Orientation.* Washington, DC: American Psychological Association.

American Psychological Association. (2011). *APA Policy Statements on Lesbian, Gay, and Bisexual and Transgender Concerns.* Washington, DC: American Psychological Association, 1–38.

Arndt, M., and De Bruin, G. (2006). Attitudes toward lesbians and gay men relations with gender, race and religion among university students. *Psychology in Society*, 33, 16–30.

Badgett, L., Donnelly, C., and Kibbe, J. (1992). *Pervasive Patterns of Discrimination against Lesbians and Gay Men: Evidence from Surveys across the United States.* Washington, DC: National Gay & Lesbian Task Force Policy Institute.

Barrett, N., Lewis, J., and Dwyer, A. E. (2011). *Effects of Disclosure of Sexual Identity at Work for Gay, Lesbian, Bisexual, Transgender and Intersex (GLBTI) Employees in Queensland.* In Proceedings of the 25th Annual Australian and New Zealand Academy of Management Conference, Australian and New Zealand Academy of Management (ANZAM), Amora Hotel, Wellington.

Beemyn, B. G. (2003). Serving the needs of transgender college students. *Journal of Gay & Lesbian Issues in Education*, 1(1), 33–50.

Beemyn, B. G. (2005). Making campuses more inclusive of transgender students. *Journal of Gay & Lesbian Issues in Education*, 3(1), 77–87.

Beemyn, G., and Rankin, S. R. (2011). *The Lives of Transgender People*. New York, NY: Columbia University Press.

Butler, J. (1988). Performative acts and gender constitution: An essay in phenomenology and feminist theory. *Theatre Journal*, 40(4), 519–531.

Bradford, J., Ryan, C., and Rothblum, E. D. (1994). National lesbian health care survey: Implications for mental health care. *Journal of Consulting and Clinical Psychology*, 62(2), 228–242.

Braun, V., and Clarke, V. (2006). Using thematic analysis in psychology. *Qualitative Research in Psychology*, 3(2), 77–101.

Brown, R., Clarke, B., Gortmaker, V., and Robinson-Keilig, R. (2004). Assessing the campus climate for gay, lesbian, bisexual and transgender (LGBT) students using a multiple perspectives approach. *Journal of College Student Development*, 45(1), 8–26.

Browne, K. (2005). Snowball sampling: Using social networks to research non-heterosexual women. *International Journal of Social Research Methodology*, 8(1), 47–60.

Brewster, M., Velez, B., DeBlaere, C., and Moradi, B. (2012). Transgender individuals' workplace experiences: The applicability of sexual minority measures and models. *Journal of Counselling Psychology*, 59(1), 60–70.

Carr, S., and Pezzella, A. (2017). Sickness, "sin" and discrimination: Examining a challenge for UK mental health nursing practice with lesbian, gay and bisexual people. *Journal of Psychiatric and Mental Health Nursing*, 24(7), 553–560.

Chrobot-Mason, D., Button, S., and DiClementi, J. (2002). Sexual identity management strategies: An exploration of antecedents and consequences. *Sex Roles*, 45(5/6), 321–336.

Chung, Y. B. (2001). Work discrimination and coping strategies: Conceptual frameworks for counselling lesbian, gay, and bisexual clients. *The Career Development Quarterly*, 50(1), 33–44.

Cocker, C., and Hafford-Letchfield, T. (2010). Critical commentary: Out and proud? Social work's relationship with lesbian and gay equality. *British Journal of Social Work*, 40(6), 1996–2008.

Conger, J. J. (1975). Proceedings of the American Psychological Association, Incorporated, for the year 1974: Minutes of the annual meeting of the council of representatives. *American Psychologist*, 30, 620–651.

Croteau, J. M., and Lark, J. S. (1995). On being lesbian, gay, or bisexual in student affairs: A national survey of experiences on the job. *NASPA Journal*, 32(3), 189–197.

Croteau, J. M., and Von Destinon, M. (1994). A national survey of job search experiences of lesbian, gay, and bisexual student affairs professionals. *Journal of College Student Development*, 35(1), 40–45.

D'Augelli, A. R. (1989), Lesbians' and gay men's experiences of discrimination and harassment in a university community. *American Journal of Community Psychology*, 17, 317–321.

D'Augelli, A. R. (1989a). The development of a helping community for lesbians and gay men: A case study in community psychology. *Journal of Community Psychology*, 17(1), 18–29.

D'Augelli, A. R. (1989b). Gay men's and lesbian's experiences of discrimination, harassment, and indifference in a university community. *American Journal of Community Psychology*, 17(3), 317–321.

Driscoll, J. M., Kelley, F. A., and Fassinger, R. E. (1996). Relation to occupational stress and satisfaction. *Journal of Vocational Behaviour*, 48(2), 229–242.

Ellis, A. L., and Riggle, E. D. (1996). The relation of job satisfaction and degree of openness about one's sexual orientation for lesbians and gay men. *Journal of Homosexuality*, 30(2), 75–85.

Elmslie, B., and Tebaldi, E. (2007). Sexual orientation and labour market discrimination. *Journal of Labour Research*, 28(3), 436–453.

Equality Challenge Unit (2009). The experience of lesbian, gay, bisexual and trans staff and students in higher education. Research Report, London: Equality Challenge Unit.

Feinberg, L. (1999). *Transliberation: Beyond Pink and Blue*. Boston: Beacon.

Friskopp, A., and Silverstein, S. (1995). *Straight Jobs, Gay Lives*. New York: Touchstone.

Gates, T. G., and Mitchell, C. G. (2013). Workplace stigma-related experiences among lesbian, gay, and bisexual workers: Implications for social policy and practice. *Journal of Workplace Behavioral Health*, 28(3), 159–171.

Giuffre, P., Dellinger, K., and Williams, C. L. (2008). No retribution for being gay? Inequality in gay-friendly workplaces. *Sociological Spectrum*, 28(3), 254–277.

Gonsiorek, J. C., and Rudolph, J. R. (1991). Homosexual identity: Coming out and other developmental events. In Gonsiorek, J. C., and Weinrich, J. D. (eds.), *Homosexuality: Research Implications for Public Policy*. Sage, 161–176.

Gonsiorek, J. C. (1991). The empirical basis for the demise of the illness model of homosexuality. In Gonsiorek, J. C., and Weinrich, J. D. (eds.), *Homosexuality: Research Implications for Public Policy*. Sage, 115–136.

Gordon, A. R., and Meyer, I. H. (2008). Gender nonconformity as a target of prejudice, discrimination, and violence against LGB individuals. *Journal of LGBT Health Research*, 3(3), 55–71.

Hafford-Letchfield, T. (2011). Sexuality and women in care organisations: Negotiating boundaries within a gendered cultural script. In Dunk-West, P., and Hafford-Letchfield, T. (eds.) *Sexual Identities and Sexuality in Social Work: Research and Reflections from Women in the Field*. Ashgate, 11–30.

Hafford-Letchfield, T., Pezzella, A., Cole, L., and Manning, R. (2017). Transgender students in post-compulsory education: A systematic review. *International Journal of Educational Research*, 86, 1–12.

Harbeck, K. M. (1997). *Gay and Lesbian Educators: Personal Freedoms, Public Constraints*. Malden, MA: Amethyst Press and Productions.

Herek, G. M. (1984). Beyond "Homophobia". *Journal of Homosexuality*, 10(1–2), 1–21.

Herek, G. M. (1988). 'Heterosexuals' attitudes toward lesbians and gay men: Correlates and gender differences.' *The Journal of Sex Research*, 25(4), 451–477.

Herek, G. M. (2007). Confronting sexual stigma and prejudice: Theory and practice. *Journal of Social Issues*, 63(4), 905–925.

Herek, G. M. (2009). Sexual stigma and sexual prejudice in the United States: A conceptual framework. In Hope, D. A. (ed.), *Nebraska Symposium on Motivation*: Vol. 54: Contemporary perspectives on lesbian, gay, and bisexual identities. New York: Springer, 65–111.

Herek, G. M., Gillis, J. R., and Cogan, J. C. (2009). Internalized stigma among sexual minority adults: Insights from a social psychological perspective. *Journal of Counselling Psychology*, 56(1), 32.

Huebner, D. M., Rebchook, G. M., and Kegeles, S. M. (2004). Experiences of harassment, discrimination, and physical violence among young gay and bisexual men. *American Journal of Public Health*, 94(7), 1200–1203.

Iconis, R. (2010). Reducing homophobia within the college community. *Contemporary Issues in Educational Research*, 3, 67–70.

Jordan, K. M., and Deluty, R. H. (1998). Coming out for lesbian women. *Journal of Homosexuality*, 35(2), 41–63.

Juul, T., and Repa, T. (1993). A survey to examine the relationship of the openness of self-identified lesbian, gay male, and bisexual public school teachers to job stress and job satisfaction. Paper presented at the annual meeting of the American Educational Research Association, Atlanta, Ga.

Kelly, E., and Dobbin, F. (1999). Civil rights law at work: Sex discrimination and the rise of maternity leave policies. *American Journal of Sociology*, 105(2), 455–492.

Kertzner, R. M., Meyer, I. H., Frost, D. M., and Stirratt, M. J. (2009). Social and psychological wellbeing in lesbians, gay men, and bisexuals: The effects of race, gender, age, and sexual identity. *American Journal of Orthopsychiatry*, 79(4), 500–510.

King, E. B., and Cortina, J. M. (2010). The social and economic imperative of lesbian, gay, bisexual, and transgendered supportive organizational policies. *Industrial and Organizational Psychology*, 3(1), 69–78.

Lyons, H., Brenner, B., and Fassinger, R. (2005). A multicultural test of the theory of work adjustment: Investigating the role of heterosexism and fit perceptions in the job satisfaction of lesbian, gay, and bisexual employees. *Journal of Counselling Psychology*, 52(4), 537–548.

Martin, Hillias J., and Murdock, James R. (2007). *Serving Lesbian, Gay, Bisexual, Transgender, and Questioning Teens: A How-to-Do-It Manual for Librarians*. New York/London: Neal-Schuman Publishers.

McDermott, E. (2006). Surviving in dangerous places: Lesbian identity performances in the workplace, social class and psychological health. *Feminism and Psychology Journal*, 16(2), 193–211.

Meyer, I. H. (2003). Prejudice, social stress, and mental health in lesbian, gay, and bisexual populations: Conceptual issues and research evidence. *Psychological Bulletin*, 129, 674–697.

Morris, J. F., Waldo, C. R., and Rothblum, E. D. (2001). A model of predictors and outcomes of outness among lesbian and bisexual women. *American Journal of Orthopsychiatry*, 71(1), 61–71.

Pascoe, E. A., and Smart Richman, L. (2009). Perceived discrimination and health: A meta-analytic review. *Psychological Bulletin*, 135(4), 531.

Pezzella, A. (2016). Coming out in the workplace and its impact on Mental Health: Experiences of staff working in HEIs. Presented at the LGBTQ inclusivity in higher education: 1st international conference, 15th and 16th September, University of Birmingham, UK

Pitts, M., Smith, A., Mitchell, A., and Patel, S. (2006). Private lives: A report on the health and wellbeing of GLBTI Australians. *Australian Research Centre in Sex, Health and Society*. Melbourne, VIC: La Trobe University.

Powers, B., and Ellis, A. (1995). *A Manager's Guide to Sexual Orientation in the Workplace*. London/New York: Routhledge.

Ragins, B., Singh, R., and Cornwell, J. (2007). Making the invisible visible: Fear and disclosure of sexual orientation at work. *Journal of Applied Psychology*, 92(4), 1103–1118.

Riggle, E. D., Whitman J. S., Olson, A., Rostosky, S. S., and Strong, S. (2008). The positive aspects of being a lesbian or gay man. *Professional Psychology: Research and Practice*, 39(2), 210–217.

Rostosky, S. S., and Riggle, E. (2002). 'Out' at work: The relation of actor and partner workplace policy and internalized homophobia to disclosure status. *Journal of Counselling Psychology*, 49 (4), 411–419.

Rumens, N., and Kerfoot, D. (2009). Gay men at work: (Re) constructing the self as professional. *Human Relations*, 62(5), 763–786.

Schmitt, J. P., and Kurdek, L. A. (1985). Age and gender differences in and personality correlates of loneliness in different relationships. *Journal of Personality Assessment*, 49(5), 485–496.

Sharpe, S. (2002). 'It's just hard to come to terms with': Young people's views on homosexuality. *Sex Education*, 2(3), 263–277.

Smith, N. J., Wright, T., Reilly, C., and Esposito, J. (2008). A national study of LGBT educators' perceptions of their workplace climate. Paper Presented at the Annual Conference of the American Educational Research Association, New York.

Subhrajit, C. (2014). Problems faced by LGBT people in the mainstream society: some recommendations. *International Journal of Interdisciplinary and Multidisciplinary Studies*, 1(5), 317–331.

Stonewall (2013). *LGBT in Britain: Lesbian, Gay and Bisexual People's Experiences and Expectations of Discrimination*. London: Stonewall.

Stonewall (2014). *Workplace Equality Index 2014*. London: Stonewall.

Stonewall (2017). *LGBT in Britain: Hate Crime and Discrimination*. London: Stonewall.

Valentine, D. (2007). *Imagining Transgender: An Ethnography of a Category*. Durham, NC: Duke University Press.

Williams, C. L., Giuffre, P. A., and Dellinger, K. (2009). The gay-friendly closet. *Sexuality Research and Social Policy*, 6(1), 29–45.

8 Measuring relationship quality in an international study

Exploratory and confirmatory factor validity[1]

Jill M. Chonody, Jacqui Gabb, Mike Killian and Priscilla Dunk-West

Introduction

This study reports on the operationalisation and testing of the newly developed Relationship Quality (RQ) scale, designed to assess an individual's perception of his or her RQ in their current partnership. Methods: Data were generated through extended sampling from an original UK-based research project, *Enduring Love? Couple relationships in the 21st century*. This mixed methods study was designed to investigate how couples experience, understand and sustain their long-term relationships. This article utilises the cross-sectional, community sample ($N = 8,132$) from this combined data set, drawn primarily from the United Kingdom, United States, and Australia. A two-part approach to scale development was employed. An initial 15-item pool was subjected to exploratory factor analysis leading into confirmatory factor analysis using structural equation modeling. Results: The final 9-item scale evidenced convergent construct validity and known-groups validity along with strong reliability. Conclusion: Implications for future research and professional practice are discussed.

Even though divorce is commonplace and many couples choose to live together without marrying, romantic coupling is a patterned and predictable feature of adulthood. This coupling has significant implications beyond the relationship, including personal emotional well-being (e.g. Proulx, Helms & Buehler, 2007) and physical health (e.g. Kiecolt-Glaser & Newton, 2001). Understanding how individuals create enduring coupledom is, therefore, important for both research and practice, and measuring relationship quality (RQ) is an essential aspect. As such, the study of relationship satisfaction has a long history in the substantive literature. Many of the existing scales in this area are problem focused and/or validated with a sample of couples engaged in therapy. These scales may serve a specific function, but we sought to create an alternative—a *strengths-based approach* to the measurement of RQ. In other words, our aim was to develop a scale that measures the *positive* aspects of a relationship, namely, RQ, using a large international diverse community sample.

In our definition of RQ, we do not presuppose that couples are "happy" or that their relationships are trouble-free; however, we start from the premise that these partnerships are "working" at an emotional and/or practical level (Gabb & Fink, 2015a) in ways that meet the needs and/or expectations of the couple. RQ thus defined draws on ideas of emotion work and working relationships within systemic psychotherapy wherein emotions have been seen as relational, embodied and culturally determined (Bertrando, 2008), and are understood as relational and performative (Fredman, 2004) rather than located within individuals. This connects with sociologically informed theorising which suggests that couples relate to and interact with each other within dynamic and intersecting micro and macro networks of relations (Burkitt, 2014) through everyday relationship practices (Gabb & Fink, 2015b).

RQ is often used interchangeably with relationship/marital satisfaction and is perhaps the most studied element of intimate relationships (Graham, Diebels & Barnow, 2011; Heyman, Sayers & Bellack, 1994). Research indicates that RQ, satisfaction and adjustment are all highly correlated, indicating that these are perhaps aspects of one latent construct (Fincham & Bradbury, 1987). Clarity of terms is crucial for research given that it is difficult to ensure that a latent construct has truly been captured when it is conflated with other, albeit similar, constructs. Delineation of an operational definition coupled with rigorous psychometric testing can advance a new scale for this substantive domain. Most existing scales, however, have failed to define their latent construct (Fincham & Bradbury, 1987; Sabatelli, 1988; Vaughn & Baier, 1999) before proceeding with scale development procedures, often drawing on items from widely used scales.

Further conceptual delimitation is, therefore, necessary to improve precision in measurement (Fincham & Bradbury, 1987; Walker & Luszcz, 2009). In addition to operationalisation, other conceptual and methodological weaknesses are found in the most commonly used scales; these are discussed in detail subsequently. After the review of relationship satisfaction/ quality scales, the process of scale development is outlined with specific reference to RQ. Our new instrument was tested with a community sample using a two-part approach, which involved both exploratory (EFA) and confirmatory (CFA) factor analyses. Results are presented, indicating the strength and reliability of this instrument. The final scale is provided for further validation alongside implications for future research and professional practice.

Review of scales

According to Graham et al. (2011) and Funk and Rogge (2007), The Locke-Wallace Marital Adjustment Test (MAT), the Kansas Marital Satisfaction Scale (KMSS), the Quality of Marriage Index (QMI), the Relationship Assessment Scale (RAS), and Karney and Bradbury's (1997) semantic differential scale are the most commonly used relationship satisfaction scales. Graham et al. (2001) also included the Marital Opinion Questionnaire (Huston & Vangelisti, 1991) and the Couples Satisfaction Index (CSI) while Funk and Rogge identified the Dyadic Assessment Scale. These scales are reviewed here to illustrate areas for measurement improvement for this substantive domain. Karney and Bradbury's semantic differential along with the Marital Opinion Questionnaire are not reviewed because these scales ask participants to rate their relationship using a series of reflective adjectives (e.g. good/bad and pleasant/unpleasant). As such, semantic differentials are substantively different from scales based on item development representing a latent construct. Thus, our review is limited to those scales that utilise a Likert-type response to a series of statements aimed at evaluating the relationship.

Locke–Wallace MAT

One of the most often cited measures for marital satisfaction (Funk & Rogge, 2007) is the Locke–Wallace MAT (Locke & Wallace, 1959). This 15-item scale asks participants to rate nine items for the level of agreement that occurs between the participant and his or her partner (e.g. philosophy of life), and a further six items are posed as questions (sample item: "Do you ever wish you had not married?"). All of the items for this scale were gleaned from previously published marital adjustment scales, and thus no specific operational definition was utilised. Instead, Locke and Wallace created this scale by choosing those items that "had the highest level of discrimination in the original studies... and would cover the important areas of marital adjustment and prediction as judged by the authors" (p. 252). This approach to scale development limits the conceptualisation to one that is purely statistical in nature.

The first nine items are on the same six-point Likert-type scale, but the final six questions each have their own response options ranging from two to four. This inconsistent scaling of the items may be problematic in terms of tau equivalent (see Graham et al., 2011, for further details) as well as weighting (Norton, 1983). Furthermore, initial validation of the scale was based on a sample of 236 participants who were "young, native-white, educated, Protestant, white-collar and professional, urban group" (Locke & Wallace, 1959, p. 254). Greater diversity in sampling strengthens scale development in terms of potential applicability to a wider range of participants.

The MAT is one of the early attempts at systematic measurement of relationship satisfaction, but despite its previous widespread use in the literature, interest in this scale is waning (Graham et al., 2011). In part, this may be due to largely outdated item content, which is not appropriate for contemporary participants. For example, Sabatelli (1988) notes that an item dealing with companionship requires a respondent to engage in all outside interests with his or her partner to achieve the highest adjustment score.

Furthermore, Graham and colleagues' meta-analysis of reliability generalisation found that the MAT was the weakest among the scales that they
assessed (see above for the complete list) at 0.785. This reliability coefficient (based on 639 reliability coefficients) is significantly lower than the
Cronbach's a reported in the original report (0.90).

Dyadic adjustment scale (DAS)

The DAS (Spanier, 1976) is a 32-item scale designed to measure marital
quality or RQ among long-term couples and is also widely used in the literature (Funk & Rogge, 2007). Like the MAT, item development for this scale
was based on scales available at the time, and prior to data collection, items
were reviewed before the final item pool were factor analyzed to create the
scale. While Spanier does include an operational definition for dyadic adjustment, the items were still drawn from known scales.

Given Spanier's approach, 12 of the 15 items from the MAT are
included on the DAS (Funk & Rogge, 2007). Some of these items are
simply outdated. For example, one item inquires about the degree to
which the couple agrees on "conventionality", defined parenthetically
as "correct or proper behavior". For contemporary participants, and a
diversely constituted sample, understandings of "correct" or "proper"
behaviour are unlikely to be universal. Furthermore, the reliance on the
MAT fails to address the problem of inconsistent weighting of items and
conceptual overlap between relationship concepts (Norton, 1983). Many
relational elements (e.g. finances, recreations and major decisions) are
included on the DAS, but these issues are not necessarily applicable to
all couples (i.e. noncohabiting couples). Such factors are more effectively assessed via other scales that attempt to pinpoint other relationship issues.

One of the strengths of the DAS is that this scale can be used to assess
RQ with both married and cohabiting couples. However, cohabiting couples were not included in the original sample used to test the scale. Given
that psychometric studies are sample dependent, this approach to scale development is worrisome, particularly in light of limited couple and participant diversity. The sample used to develop the DAS was White, married
individuals from working- and middle-class backgrounds. The diversity in
socio-economic sampling strengthens the potential applicability of the scale
while its racial specificity is delimiting.

Due to its evidence of good reliability and factor structure, its popularity among researchers is understandable. The reported Cronbach's
a in the original study was 0.96. A large coefficient such as this suggests that there may be item redundancy in the scale, which inflates the
correlations between items. Scale length may also be contributing to
this coefficient, and at 32-items, some further reduction of items seems
warranted.

KMSS

KMSS (Schumm, Nichols, Schectman & Grigsby, 1983) was originally developed in the late 1970s as three single-item indicators, but subsequent data collection and analyses suggested that these items could be combined to create a general MSS. These items ask participants to rate "how satisfied are you with… your husband [wife] as a spouse?; your marriage?; and your relationship with your husband [wife]?" (Schumm et al., 1983, p. 569). In Graham et al.'s (2011) recent meta-analyses of reliability generalisation, researchers found that the KMSS was the strongest among the scales assessed, with a Cronbach's a that averaged 0.95. Schumm et al. (1983) report inter-item correlations between 0.93 and 0.95, and these high correlations suggest item redundancy as does the nearly perfect Cronbach's a. Nonetheless, the KMSS exhibits good face validity and has been found to be related to other satisfaction instruments (see Graham et al., 2011). Its brevity is also a significant advantage, allowing it to be readily included alongside other relationship instruments. It addresses the issue of conceptual overlap between relationship satisfaction and relationship issues that may influence satisfaction (e.g. division of labour); however, as it was originally written, the items are geared toward marital relationships and its applicability to unmarried couples is thus limited.

QMI

The QMI (Norton, 1983) is a six-item scale that measures "the goodness of the relationship gestalt." Items include "We have a good marriage" and "Our marriage is strong" (Norton, 1983, p. 143). As mentioned above, the use of the terms "marriage/marital" in the items is problematic for researchers who seek to be more inclusive in their sampling frames. However, Norton took a rigorous approach to the development of the QMI and sought to tackle problems found in the existing scales. Specifically, Norton aimed to eliminate the conceptual overlap between RQ and *components* of a relationship that can impact RQ. Additionally, Norton clearly delineated a definition for RQ and how it should be captured, as evaluative not descriptive. In other words, Norton proposed that relationships can be *described* by a set of qualities or the relationship can be *evaluated* (i.e. is this relationship good?).

While Norton's operational definition guided his decision-making process, the items for the QMI were part of another scale, the Partner Communication Scale. Twenty of the 261 items on this scale were found to "loosely satisfy the criteria of evaluative" (p. 144). Once the data were collected, the items were subjected to a two-stage process of reduction. First, a correlational analysis was performed, then a factor analysis. In Graham et al.'s (2011) reliability analyses, the QMI was found to exhibit strong reliability (0.94). But there is inconsistent scaling across the items in the QMI, with five items being assessed on a 7-point scale and one global item (overall happiness with marriage) evaluated on a 10-point scale. In sum, the primary drawback of this scale is that the terminology is limiting. It also needs further testing to determine its applicability with a diverse sample, as the original sample was drawn from the Midwest without socio-demographic information on education, race/ethnicity, religion or sexual orientation being provided.

RAS

The RAS (Hendrick, 1988) is a seven-item scale designed to measure satisfaction in general. Sample items include "How good is your relationship compared to most?" and "How many problems are there in your relationship?". The RAS aimed to address item content that was delineated by marital status, something that was common in standardised scales at the time. Hendrick previously tested five of the seven items with married couples in another study, and the full RAS was then later psychometrically tested with undergraduate students enrolled in a psychology class. Only responses from students who reported that they were "in love" were retained for further analyses ($n = 125$). Factor analysis of these data indicated a strong factor structure. A second study was then undertaken with 57 dating couples attending the university who were given course credit or a small stipend for participation. No information is given about the socio-demographic composition of the sample.

The RAS correlates with the DAS showing evidence of concurrent validity, and reliability was good (0.86). However, some of the items appear problematic given the focus of this scale is RQ. For example, one item reads, "To what extent has your relationship met your original expectations?" This item does not appear to have face validity, given that an individual could justifiably indicate that this relationship does not meet his or her original expectations, yet the *quality* of the relationship may be very high. Furthermore, items that invite comparisons to others, such as "how good is your relationship compared to most?" presuppose a normative underlying concept and a shared understanding of what constitutes a "good relationship."

CSI

Utilising factor analysis and item response theory (IRT), Funk and Rogge (2007) developed three versions (32-, 16-, and 4-items) of the CSI. IRT allows researchers to determine which items are providing the most information, thus identifying items that are more precise in their measurement. The CSI is the only instrument to take this approach (Graham et al., 2011). Once again, previous scales on relationship satisfaction were used to create this "new" scale, and an operational definition for the latent construct was not provided. Instead, all of the items from these scales were included, aside from redundancies. An additional 71 further items were included, 25 items selected from other scales of relationship satisfaction and 46 new items, of which 35 items were "written from scratch" and the remaining 11 were modified items from the MAT and the DAS. No further information is provided on how the new items were written.

Evidence of convergent construct validity was demonstrated for the CSI suggesting that it is measuring the construct of satisfaction as conceptualised by past scale developments. Relatedly, reliability was quite high at 0.98, again raising concerns regarding item redundancies, but subsequent reports indicate lower as (0.90–0.92; Graham et al., 2011). A large ($N = 5,315$) and diverse sample (including people of colour, a range of educational backgrounds and dating couples) was obtained to test the items for the CSI, which is a significant strength; however, the lack of conceptualisation of the latent construct prior to item construction may be problematic when pinpointing what the summary scores are representing. Moreover, given that Funk and Rogge used previously developed scales, some of the items mentioned in the previous sections as potentially problematic are also found in this scale (e.g. "To what extent has your relationship met your original expectations?"). Like the MAT and DAS, some items use different types of response options; nevertheless, all of the items are placed on a five-point scale, which eliminates the weighting issue.

Summary

The most salient issue across nearly all of the scales reviewed is that the item content is not specific to the domain of relationship satisfaction or quality. Most of these scales conflate a number of relationship constructs in that item content contains aspects of relationships that may pertain to quality, but are not a *measure* of quality, an issue that has been raised in the literature for many years (e.g. Sabatelli, 1988). For example, communication influences the quality of the relationship, but is not a determinant of it (Norton, 1983). To address this issue, our scale limits the definition of RQ to those key elements that represent overall quality. In other words, relationship issues, such as division of labour within the household, are excluded from operationalisation given that these issues can be assessed by other means to determine their role, if any, in explaining RQ. This creates a conceptually clean scale with the sole focus on RQ in and of itself.

Based on our review of commonly used RQ scales, four other important issues were identified as areas of potential improvement for development of a new scale. First, lack of an operational definition that specifically articulates the focus of the scale is a key limitation. A clear conceptual definition that guides item development contributes to a parsimonious scale. As suggested above, relationship satisfaction and RQ are likely to share essential components, but further research is required to establish the precise demarcation of terms, and testing to determine the exact nature of the associations between similar latent constructs.

Second, lack of diversity in the sample used for scale validation is problematic for contemporary studies. The inclusion of racial/ethnically diverse samples as well as couples who represent modern day intimacies, including residency (e.g. cohabitating and living-apart-together relationships) and sexuality (same-sex, bisexual and opposite-sex couples). These are important features for a scale that is meant to be representative and/or reflect community-wide diversity. Same-sex couples and cohabitators are increasingly more salient for research foci, yet available scales may not be appropriately designed to be inclusive of such diverse relationships (Graham et al., 2011).

Third, the use of the word "marital" or "marriage" in the items is problematic because these items are thus not inclusive of other coupled relationships, including those who are in a domestic partnership, civil union or de facto relationship. Changes to currently used scales may need further psychometric testing to determine their usefulness with other populations (see Graham et al., 2011, for information on reliability of scales with different couple types). Finally, many of these scales are quite long. Respondent burden and relevance of item content are both important features in research that endeavors to inform practice and advance the substantive knowledge base.

Current study

To address the weaknesses identified in the above scales, we sought to develop a new scale to measure RQ. Based on our review of the literature, we operationalised the construct of RQ, and then proceeded to test our items, both with experts and through advanced statistical analysis. Our primary goal was to create a strengths-based scale that addressed limitations in the currently available scales that are related to RQ, including the recruitment of a diverse, international sample.

Method

Item development

Based on the literature, RQ was operationalised as the degree to which a commitment exists, mutual enjoyment (including companionship) is present and a sense that this person is the "right" one. To that end, 26 items that were geared toward these constructs were written; 13 were oriented toward commitment and companionship and the other 13 covered RQ as it relates to one's relationship with his or her partner (e.g. "My partner is usually aware of my needs"). Items were designed to interrogate the ways in which partnerships are sustained through ordinary (Brownlie, 2014) everyday relationship work (Gabb & Fink, 2015a), drawing on UK sociological analysis that has advanced a "practices approach" to study families (Morgan, 1996, 2011), intimacy (Jamieson, 1998) and personal life (Smart, 2007). This ongoing relationship work sustains RQ and maintains coupledom.

The initial study (*Enduring Love? Couple relationships in the 21st century* [RES-062-23-3056] was funded by the Economic and Social Research Council and completed in the UK) was designed in dialogue with members of a Strategy Board, including policy makers, professional practitioners and senior researchers. At the outset of the project, interviews were completed with key stakeholders in UK family and relationship support services and government departments. Drafts of the survey were subsequently circulated among the Strategy Board and the research community more widely. This enabled us to edit and add items and refine the survey instrument. This aimed to ensure that the items were attentive to the concerns of relationship support organisations and the needs of adult couples (Walker, Barrett, Wilson & Chang, 2010) and that findings would provide potentially useful information on how individuals experience and perceive their coupledom.

Web-based surveys have quickly moved from "novel idea to routine use" (Dillman, Smyth & Christian, 2007, p. 447). Online surveys allow for a diverse and international group of individuals to be sampled and can capture opinions on RQ from a wide spectrum of people. This has the capacity to generate high-quality data (e.g. Chang & Krosnick, 2009; Gosling, Vazire, Srivastava & John, 2004). Good practice guidelines for Internet-mediated research (IMR) are becoming well established (e.g. Hewson, 2003; Hewson & Laurent, 2012) and our survey was developed in line with these protocols. We also consulted with an online survey expert to make sure the instrument was technically and ethically robust, in accordance with the British Psychological Society guidelines, and that items were not double barreled or difficult to interpret.

In response to all of the above consultation, some items were reworked or replaced. These 26 reformulated items were used in our survey of couples to measure RQ; however, one item ("Raising children together makes our relationship stronger") was not used in any of the RQ analyses given that it does not apply to all survey participants. Items utilised a five-point Likert-type scale (1 = *strongly disagree* and 5 = *strongly agree*).

Data collection

Data were collected in two waves via anonymous online surveys on *Survey Monkey* as part of a larger survey on enduring coupledom. In Wave 1, survey administration was targeted at a UK sample. Advantages of IMR methods include the capacity to recruit participants irrespective of their geographical location, and the ability to target specialist and/or "hard-to-reach" populations. Survey participants were recruited through features and news coverage of the research project posted on various online forums, newsletters and community group noticeboards, especially those clustered around parenting and relationship support.

In Wave 2, the survey was replicated in the United States and Australia. However, recruitment in these two countries remained limited and as such there were smaller samples here than those obtained in the UK data collection phase. The primary method for recruitment in the United States and Australia was snowballing techniques that relied on sharing the survey link with interested participants, alongside posts (and reposts) made on Twitter and Facebook, as well through university networks where the researchers worked.

Once missing data were removed (i.e. those who opened the survey but did not complete any items) along with respondents not in a relationship (e.g. divorced), the final sample (N = 8,132) was obtained. While the study focused on long-term enduring relationships, what constitutes "long-term" was not specified because pilot research indicated that couples' perception of relationship duration is informed by age, childhood, personal relationship biographies and an imagined future in this relationship (Gabb & Fink, 2015a). That is to say, perceptions of relationship duration are relative.

The survey items that were utilised in this study, in addition to the RQ scale, are described below along with the hypotheses related to their inclusion. Other survey questions were included in the questionnaire, but were not used in the current analysis; these are thus described elsewhere.

Convergent construct validity variable. A single-item indicator was used to determine overall *happiness with one's relationship*, and as a test of convergent construct validity. Participants were asked to rate this question: "How happy are you with your relationship overall?" employing a five-point Likert-type scale (1 = *very unhappy* and 5 = *very happy*). We hypothesised a positive correlation between this single item and the RQ scale.

Known-groups validity variables. Gender included "male, female, and other" and was used as a test of known-groups validity. Substantive literature indicates that gender is not related to relationship satisfaction (Jackson, Miller, Oka & Henry, 2014); thus, we anticipated no significant difference in RQ for this variable. *Parenthood* was assessed by a dichotomous question ("yes/no") and used as another test of known groups. A meta-analysis of the role of parenthood in relationship satisfaction indicated that parents are less satisfied than nonparents (Twenge, Campbell & Foster, 2003). Therefore, we hypothesised that parents would indicate less RQ than nonparents.

Socio-demographic variables. A number of other socio-demographic variables were also included and descriptively used in this study. *Age* was measured categorically ("16–24, 25–34, 35–44, 45–54, 55–64, and 65+"). *Sexual orientation* included "heterosexual, gay/lesbian, bisexual, and other." *Religious affiliation* comprised all major religions as well as the opportunity to add one that was not listed. *Education* was measured categorically according to country-specific educational standards. Some of these categories were then combined to create a description of the overall sample. *Employment* was measured categorically and then later combined to create a description. *Relationship status* was measured as "married, living together, not living together, domestic partner, and dating." The *length of the relationship* was measured categorically ("under 1 year, 1–5 years, 6–10 years,

11–15 years, 16–20 years, and 20þ years"). *Past use of relationship support* (e.g. counseling with a therapist or pastor/religious leader, seeking consultation with a primary care physician/general practitioner) was a dichotomous question ("yes/no").

Data analysis

Demographic characteristics reported by respondents indicate a diverse and multinational sample of individuals (Table 8.1). Approximately 12% of the sample identified as a sexual minority, nearly 50% reported being either Atheist or Agnostic and 25% of participants were not married, but rather were living together/in a civil union. However, the sample was also highly educated (75.7% with a university degree) and the most frequent response for length of relationship was over 20 years (mode with 30.6% of responses). The race and ethnicity characteristics of respondents are provided in Table 8.2 and demonstrate the complex nature of this international sample of individuals. From the total sample across all countries, around 25% of respondents reported their race/ethnicity as Black, Asian or biracial/mixed ethnicity.

Evaluating item performance

Measures of central tendency were checked prior to undertaking the analysis of the factor structure for the RQ scale. Skew and kurtosis were not greater than 2.5 on any item, and variance in responses was acceptable. As a result of this evaluation, no items were removed.

Next, bivariate correlations between all of the items were performed to determine the degree to which these items were related to one another. No items were found to exceed a correlation of 0.90 (range of $r = 0.081$ to $r = 0.644$, all $p < 0.001$); however, 10 items were found to have no correlations > 0.30, indicating that the item had a weak relationship with the other items. These items were removed, and the remaining 15 items were utilised for the EFA.

EFA

The overall sample ($N = 8,132$) was split randomly and equally into two subsamples (Table 8.1). The two subsamples significantly differed only by gender ($\chi^2 = 4.13$, $df = 1$, $p = 0.42$), with a greater proportion of women in the EFA subsample ($n = 3,203$, 81.7% vs. $n = 3,161$, 79.9% in the CFA subsample). This difference between the two subsamples was deemed negligible, and there were no other significant differences between groups by demographic variables ($p > 0.05$). Split-half validation was then conducted on the two separate samples of 4,066 respondents using first EFA and then CFA. The sub-sample for the EFA contained 3,675 complete responses across the initial

Table 8.1 Socio-demographic description of sample

Variable	Total sample, n = 8,132	EFA half, n = 4,066	CFA half, n = 4,066
Gender			
Male	1516 (19.2%)	719 (18.3%)	797 (20.1%)
Female	6364 (80.8%)	3203 (81.7%)	3161 (79.9%)
Age			
16–24	631 (8.0%)	310 (7.8%)	321 (8.1%)
25–34	2177 (27.5%)	1099 (27.8%)	1078 (27.2%)
35–44	2023 (25.5%)	1014 (25.7%)	1009 (25.4%)
45–54	1565 (19.8%)	733 (19.6%)	792 (20.0%)
55–64	1116 (14.1%)	546 (13.8%)	570 (14.4%)
65+	409 (5.2%)	210 (5.3%)	199 (5.0%)
Sexual orientation			
Heterosexual	6839 (88.0%)	3405 (88.0%)	3434 (87.9%)
Gay/lesbian	499 (6.4%)	247 (6.4%)	252 (6.5%)
Bisexual	437 (5.6%)	219 (5.6%)	218 (5.6%)
Country			
United Kingdom	5683 (69.9%)	2837 (69.8%)	2846 (70.0%)
United States	1652 (20.3%)	820 (20.2%)	832 (20.5%)
Australia	491 (6.0%)	255 (6.3%)	236 (3.7%)
Other country	306 (3.8%)	154 (3.8%)	152 (3.7%)
Education level			
No high school diploma	102 (1.5%)	46 (1.4%)	56 (1.7%)
High school diploma/ equivalency	309 (4.6%)	163 (4.9%)	146 (4.3%)
Vocational training/some college	1227 (18.2%)	598 (17.8%)	629 (18.6%)
Professional/bachelor's degree	2855 (42.3%)	1434 (42.7%)	1421 (41.9%)
Master's/PhD	2257 (33.4%)	1119 (33.3%)	1138 (33.6%)
Employment			
Part-time work	1796 (26.4%)	894 (26.3%)	902 (26.4%)
Full-time work	3143 (46.2%)	1540 (45.3%)	1603 (47.0%)
Retired	503 (7.4%)	256 (7.5%)	247 (7.2%)
Homemaker/carer	519 (7.6%)	256 (7.5%)	263 (7.7%)
Volunteer	85 (1.2%)	51 (1.5%)	34 (1.0%)
Full/part-time student	454 (6.7%)	237 (7.0%)	217 (6.4%)
Not employed or working	180 (2.6%)	102 (3.0%)	78 (2.3%)
Disabled	129 (1.9%)	60 (1.8%)	69 (2.0%)
Religious affiliation			
Christian (Protestant, Catholic)	2976 (46.7%)	1479 (46.8%)	1497 (46.5%)
Jewish	111 (1.7%)	51 (1.6%)	60 (0.5%)
Muslim	53 (0.8%)	28 (0.9%)	25 (0.8%)
Buddhist	81 (1.3%)	47 (1.5%)	34 (1.1%)
None	3118 (48.9%)	1534 (48.6%)	1584 (49.3%)
Other (Sikh, Hindu)	34 (0.5%)	18 (0.6%)	16 (0.5%)
Parent (yes)	2966 (44.4%)	1477 (44.3%)	1489 (44.4%)

(Continued)

Table 8.1 (Continued)

Variable	Total sample, n = 8,132	EFA half, n = 4,066	CFA half, n = 4,066
Relationship status			
Married	4981 (62.7%)	2500 (63.1%)	2481 (62.3%)
Couple- not living together	832 (10.5%)	406 (10.3%)	426 (10.7%)
Living together	1744 (22.0%)	859 (21.7%)	885 (22.2%)
Civil partnership	250 (3.1%)	129 (3.3%)	121 (3.0%)
Dating	133 (1.7%)	65 (1.6%)	68 (1.7%)
Number of years in relationship			
Under 1 year	336 (4.2%)	169 (4.2%)	167 (4.2%)
1–5	1813 (22.6%)	915 (22.8%)	898 (22.4%)
6–10	1506 (18.8%)	746 (18.6%)	760 (18.9%)
11–15	1133 (14.1%)	567 (14.2%)	566 (14.1%)
16–20	779 (9.7%)	384 (9.6%)	395 (9.8%)
20+	2451 (30.6%)	1224 (30.6%)	1227 (30.6%)
Relationship support (no)	4775 (65.7%)	2372 (65.2%)	2403 (66.2%)
Happy with relationship[b]	4.29 (0.87)	4.28 (0.86)	4.30 (0.87)
Relationship quality[c]	37.70 (5.97)	37.63 (5.94)	37.79 (6.01)

[a]Sample sizes are different on each variable due to missing data.
[b]Theoretical range = 1–5.
[c]Theoretical range = 9–45 (based on final scale).

Table 8.2 Ethnicity by country

Ethnicity	Total N	Country of respondent			
		UK	USA	AUS	Other
White British, American, Australian	5004 (74.3%)	3874 (81.5%)	670 (49.2%)	393 (97.3%)	67 (30.9%)
Other White	1286 (19.1%)	601 (12.6%)	561 (41.2%)	5 (1.2%)	119 (54.8%)
Caribbean	29 (0.4%)	23 (0.5%)	4 (0.3%)	5 (1.2%)	2 (0.9%)
African/African American	69 (1.0%)	41 (0.9%)	27 (2.0%)	0 (0.0%)	1 (0.5%)
Other African decent	11 (0.2%)	5 (0.1%)	6 (0.4%)	0 (0.0%)	0 (0.0%)
Indian, Asian subcontinent	63 (0.9%)	53 (1.1%)	5 (0.4%)	0 (0.0%)	5 (2.3%)
Asian	64 (1.0%)	36 (0.8%)	17 (1.2%)	1 (0.2%)	10 (4.6%)
Hispanic/Latino	18 (0.3%)	0 (0.0%)	17 (1.2%)	0 (0.0%)	1 (0.5%)
Native/ Aboriginal	5 (0.1%)	0 (0.0%)	2 (0.1%)	3 (0.7%)	0 (0.0%)
Mixed ethnicity, other	186 (2.8%)	119 (2.5%)	53 (3.9%)	2 (0.5%)	12 (5.5%)

set of items (90.4%). Bartlett's test of sphericity (χ^2 = 20,904.61, df = 105, $p < 0.001$) and KMO's (Kaiser–Myer–Olkin) measure of sample adequacy were excellent (KMO = 0.946), and the amount of explained variance was good (50.5%). Items were removed from the model based on their factor loadings and amount of variance in the item explained by the factor model. The initial factor solution indicated two factors with 15 items; however, several items had significant loadings (>0.40) on both factors. After several iterations and removal of poor performing items as indicated by cross loadings or a weak factor loading (<0.40), a final factor model was achieved. This model contained nine items and had a Cronbach's a reliability coefficient of 0.888. Bartlett's test of sphericity (χ^2 = 14,780.16, df = 36, $p < 0.001$) and KMO's measure of sample adequacy were again excellent (KMO = 0.928), and the amount of explained variance improved (54.2%) from the initial model. Table 8.3 provides the final factor loadings and communalities for the scale.

Our data analysis plan for testing the newly developed RQ scale commenced with a review of item performance, including skew and kurtosis and a correlational analysis. Next, an EFA with SPSS 22.0 was performed to determine the factor structure of the scale, and any poorly performing items were eliminated. The EFA was conducted using principle component analysis as the extraction method, and eigenvalues greater than 1 were used to identify the factors. To improve the interpretation of the factor loadings, an orthogonal rotation was used (Varimax). A CFA using structural equation modeling with MPlus 7.3 provided the final factor structure of the scale. Modification indices generated during the CFA were considered if the modification would create a change in the model χ^2 value greater than 3.84 ($p < 0.05$), which is a statistically significant improvement in the model. Though researchers should use these post hoc modifications to the model with care, these changes can be done where supported by theory (Jackson, Gillaspy & Purc-Stephenson, 2009; Kline, 2011). The final model was then used for tests of convergent construct validity and known-groups validity.

Table 8.3 Exploratory factor analysis: factor loadings (n = 4,066)

Relationship quality item	Factor loading	Commonality score
I am content in our relationship	0.838	0.703
This is the relationship I always dreamed of	0.794	0.630
We have grown apart over time[a]	0.748	0.559
I am totally committed to making this relationship work	0.745	0.554
We enjoy each other's company	0.733	0.537
My partner is usually aware of my needs	0.706	0.499
I think of my partner as my soul mate	0.703	0.495
My partner makes me laugh	0.686	0.471
We have shared values	0.655	0.430

[a]Reverse scored.

Results

Demographics

The first wave of the survey was administered through a mixed methods study based in the UK (n = 7,654), with the subsequent wave in the United States (n = 917) and Australia (n = 465) producing additional responses. Individuals responding to the online survey across both waves included participants representing 60 different countries, including Japan, Botswana, China, Peru, India and the Dominican Republic, as well as a number of other European countries. The two waves resulted in a final sample of 8,132 individuals who fully completed the survey and reported being in a long-term relationship.

Factor Commonality with values ≥0.95 indicative of acceptable model fit (Hu & Bentler, 1999; Kline, 2011). SRMR is a measure of the residuals between the input covariance and measurement model matrices. SRMR values less than 0.08 or 0.10 indicate good model fit (Brown, 2006). Lastly, RMSEA adjusts for model parsimony and estimates the difference between model covariances and the observed covariances. Values between 0.08 and 0.10 are indicative of adequate fit. RMSEA values for each model were tested for significant differences from 0.05 along with the 90% confidence interval of the estimates (Kline, 2011).

The CFA tested the factor structure for the RQ scale found in the EFA. Initial results indicated adequate fit (see Table 8.4), but further improvements to the model were suggested through the indices produced (χ^2 > 3.84, p < 0.05). Correlations between individual item error terms were added to the model, given that they offered the greatest decrease in the model χ^2 value. Two modifications were made to the model prior to the final model. In order, the error terms for items were allowed to correlate which reduced the χ^2 by 170.35 (p < 0.001) and then by 74.85 (p < 0.001). The final model demonstrated excellent fit across all fit indices (see Table 8.4). Figure 8.1 provides the factor loadings and error terms for the final RQ scale, and Table 8.5 lists the items.

Reliability

A total RQ score was calculated by summing responses to the items identified from the EFA and CFA. The resulting measure demonstrated high internal consistency reliability.

CFA

With the other half of the sample (n = 4,066), CFA was conducted. This subsample contained 3,858 complete responses (94.8%) across the nine items identified in the EFA. The initial and final CFA models are listed in Table 8.4.

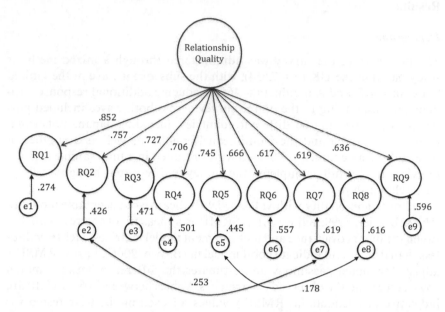

Figure 8.1 Confirmatory factor analysis: item loadings (*n* = 4,066). Items correspond to item list in Table 8.5.

Table 8.4 Confirmatory factor analysis: model fit indices (*n* = 4,066)

Model	χ^2	df	χ^2/df	RMSEA	90% CI	p-value	CFI	TLI	SRMR
Initial	594.12***	27	22.0	0.074	0.069–0.079	$p < 0.001$	0.965	0.953	0.027
Final	292.73***	25	11.7	0.053	0.047–0.058	$p = 0.199$	0.983	0.976	0.020

CFI = comparative fit index; RMSEA = root mean square error of approximation; SRMR = standardized root mean square residual; TLI = Tucker–Lewis index; χ^2 = chi-square; *df* = degrees of freedom.
***$p < 0.001$.

Table 8.5 Final relationship quality (RQ) scale

	Items
RQ1	I am content in our relationship
RQ2	This is the relationship I always dreamed of
RQ3	We have grown apart over time[a]
RQ4	I am totally committed to making this relationship work
RQ5	We enjoy each other's company
RQ6	My partner is usually aware of my needs
RQ7	I think of my partner as my soul mate
RQ8	My partner makes me laugh
RQ9	We have shared values

[a]Reverse scored.

To assess the fit of the obtained RQ data to the EFA measurement model, multiple fit indices were obtained. The model χ^2 per degrees of freedom (χ^2 df), Tucker–Lewis index (TLI), comparative fit index (CFI), standardised root mean square residual (SRMR) and the root mean square error of approximation (RMSEA) were all used. Lower scores for the model χ^2 statistic (Kline, 2011) and the model χ^2/df indicate better fit between the data and model. Bollen (1989) suggests a χ^2/df value between 2.0 and 3.0 indicates adequate model fit. The CFI and TLI compare the model to the fit of a baseline model

Consistent with the literature, parents are found to report lower relationship satisfaction (Twenge et al., 2003); thus, this finding provides evidence of known-groups validity. Last, no significant differences in RQ scores, $t = 0.31$, $df = 7,307$, $p = 0.753$, and Cohen's $d = 0.04$, were reported between men ($M = 37.76$, $SD = 5.95$) and women ($M = 37.71$, $SD = 5.98$). This is also consistent with the literature that suggests relationship satisfaction is not different by gender (Jackson et al., 2014).

Discussion and applications to practice

Results of our study provide evidence for the initial validation of the RQ scale. Designed for and tested with a sample of individuals in an enduring relationship, this new scale shows evidence of factorial validity, convergent construct validity and known-groups validity. This scale is also short and easy to administer with strong reliability. For these reasons, this scale may be useful in survey research on couple relationships. The RQ also advances contemporary research interests in diverse couples (e.g. cohabitators) using the word "partner" instead of spouse/husband/wife. This new scale builds on established measures, but avoids some of the problematic aspects of those scales, including conceptual overlap with other relationship issues, such as conflict, communication or parenthood. These variables should be studied as factors *related to* RQ instead of components *of it*. Thus, other standardised scales or single-item indicators can assess these issues to determine how other relationship issues impact overall RQ. This is an improvement over existing scales of relationship satisfaction (e.g. MAT, DAS and CSI) that conflate these concepts.

The new RQ scale also, and importantly, represents a *strengths-based approach* to the measurement of RQ in that items are focused on positive elements of the relationship instead of a problems-focused agenda. By focusing on elements of the relationship that may be working, the scale summary score is indicative of the degree to which positive aspects of the relationship are present. The focus on everyday relationship practices as the means through which couples sustain their long-term partnerships thus shifts the emphasis away from regular markers of RQ (such "good" communication or regular and mutually "enjoyable" sexual intimacy) and traditional, culturally inscribed understandings of what makes a relationship work. This has the capacity to extend understandings of how RQ is manifest, in an everyday sense, and to enrich knowledge on what constitutes RQ in a working relationship. As such, it has the potential to make a significant contribution to and have practical applications in the fields of relationship support and intervention.

Utilising a community sample, instead of one comprised of individuals/ couples engaged in relationship therapy, means that the RQ scale has the capacity to be used with a wider and/or general population. Future research would be needed to determine if it could be used specifically with those engaged in couples work. For example, given the items on the RQ scale, it may be useful as an initial assessment tool to determine where the couple presently are in their relationship, and provide some indication of where they may want to aim toward, in the future. Relatedly, future research is needed to determine if the RQ scale can discriminate between distressed and nondistressed couples; this would expand the usefulness of this scale to a clinical setting. Further exploration of the RQ scales criterion-related and construct validity may reveal clinical utility and potential uses by practitioners.

The RQ scale provides an indication of RQ at one point in time. This may be helpful for both researchers and practitioners who seek to obtain an over-all assessment of individual perceptions of relationships and determine the role of other factors that may be influencing RQ (e.g. communication). How-ever, to fully comprehend RQ, a past point of reference is necessary, and thus longitudinal data are needed to determine any change over time (Bradbury, Fincham & Beach, 2000). Future research could seek to use the RQ in longitu-dinal studies with both individuals in the community and those who are help seeking, to determine its sensitivity to changes in RQ over time.

The results of our study should be considered within the framework of its limitations. The survey was completed by respondents representing 60 different countries; however, the sample was collected primarily from three countries. The vast majority of these respondents were from Euro-centric countries with historic ties to British colonialism. Furthermore, the sample was exceedingly well educated and female. Given the online nature of the survey, a high level of education and greater participation by women can be expected. Notwithstanding these limitations, our sample did achieve some degree of diversity in terms of other socio-demographic characteristics. Just over 37% of the sample was cohabitating, in civil union/domestic partner-ship or were noncohabitating long-term partners; 12% of respondents re-ported their sexual orientation as lesbian, gay or bisexual. There was also a good distribution of age.

Generalisation of the results should be done with caution, and future re-search with the RQ scale should employ methods to obtain more diverse samples of individuals, especially in terms of education, socio-economic background and cultural diversity. The split-half factor validation process was exploratory and as such the RQ measure was first identified through EFA and later error terms were allowed to correlate in the CFA model where appropriate. Though the use of the split-half factor validation process conducted with the present sample adds confidence to the factorial validity of the RQ scale, psychometric studies are sample dependent, and additional validation studies of the RQ scale are warranted, including further investigation into how the RQ correlates to other standardised measures of relationship/marital satisfaction.

In sum, the findings from our preliminary study indicate initial validation of the RQ scale. Based on a large community-dwelling sample from multiple countries, the RQ showed good reliability and evidence of validity. The RQ addressed some limitations found in other relationship scales, such as anachronistic items, limiting terms (e.g. "marital"), inconsistency in response options and includes a focus on relationship strengths without the inclusion of additional RQs (e.g. communication). Additional psychometric studies with community samples can expand the utility of this scale, which may include application in practice as an assessment tool.

Key recommendations for applying research to professional practice

- The use of scales in the professions can help in working with couples
- The concept of relationship quality requires an understanding of the everyday practices of couples, such as 'relationship practices', and can be a useful way to understand the relationship from the client(s) perspective(s)
- Relationship quality includes not only communication but other forms of interactions and meanings
- In considering relationship quality, it is important to understand the ways in which relationships intersect with other factors, such as culture, age, religion and sexual identity and parenting, as well as social issues

Note

1 Note: this article is reproduced with permission from the following publication: Research on Social Work Practice 1–11a The Author(s) 2016 Reprints and permission: sagepub.com/journals. Permissions.nav. doi:10.1177/1049731516631120 rsw.sagepub.com.

References

Bertrando, P. (2008). Emotional dances: Therapeutic dialogues as embodied systems. *Journal of Family Therapy, 30*, 362–372.

Bollen, K. A. (1989). *Structural equations with latent variables*. New York, NY: Wiley.

Bradbury, T. N., Fincham, F. D., & Beach, S. R. H. (2000). Research on the nature and determinants of marital satisfaction: A decade in review. *Journal of Marriage and Family, 62*, 964–980.

Brown, T. A. (2006). *Confirmatory factor analysis for applied research*. New York, NY: Guilford Press.

Brownlie, J. (2014). *Ordinary relationships: A sociological study of emotions, reflexivity and culture*. Basingstoke, England: Palgrave Macmillan.

Burkitt, I. (2014). *Emotions and social relations*. London, England: Sage.

Chang, L., & Krosnick, J. A. (2009). National surveys via RDD telephone interviewing versus the internet: Comparing sample representativeness and response quality. *Public Opinion Quarterly, 73*, 641–678.

Dillman, D. A., Smyth, J. D., & Christian, L. M. (2007). *Internet, mail, and mixed-mode surveys: The tailored design method*. London, England: Wiley.

Fincham, F. D., & Bradbury, T. N. (1987). The assessment of marital quality: A reevaluation. *Journal of Marriage and the Family, 49*, 797–809.

Fredman, G. (2004). *Transforming emotion: Conversations in counselling and psychotherapy*. London, England: Whurr Publishers.

Funk, J. L., & Rogge, R. D. (2007). Testing the ruler with item response theory: Increasing precision of measurement for relationship satisfaction with the couples satisfaction index. *Journal of Family Psychology, 21*, 572–583.

Gabb, J., & Fink, J. (2015a). *Couple relationships in the 21st century*. London, England: Palgrave Macmillan.

Gabb, J., & Fink, J. (2015b). Telling moments and everyday experience: Multiple methods research on couple relationships and personal lives. *Sociology, 49*, 970–987.

Gosling, S. D., Vazire, S., Srivastava, S., & John, O. P. (2004). Should we trust web-based studies? A comparative analysis of six preconceptions about Internet questionnaires. *American Psychologist, 59*, 93–104.

Graham, J. M., Diebels, K. J., & Barnow, Z. B. (2011). The reliability of relationship satisfaction: A reliability generalization meta-analysis. *Journal of Family Psychology, 25*, 39–48.

Hendrick, S. (1988). A generic measure of relationship satisfaction. *Journal of Marriage and the Family, 50*, 93–98.

Hewson, C. (2003). Conducting research on the Internet. *The Psychologist, 16*, 290–293.

Hewson, C., & Laurent, D. (2012). Research design and tools for Internet research. In J. Hughes (Ed.), *Sage Internet research methods* (Vol. 1, pp. 165–104). London, England: Sage.

Heyman, R. E., Sayers, S. L., & Bellack, A. S. (1994). Global marital satisfaction versus marital adjustment: An empirical comparison of three measures. *Journal of Family Psychology, 8*, 432–446.

Hu, L., & Bentler, P. M. (1999). Cutoff criteria for fit indexes in covariance structure analysis: Conventional criteria versus new alternatives. *Structural Equation Modeling: A Multidisciplinary Journal, 6*, 1–55.

Huston, T. L., & Vangelisti, A. L. (1991). Socioemotional behavior and satisfaction in marital relationships: A longitudinal study. *Journal of Personality and Social Psychology, 61*, 721–733.

Jackson, D. L., Gillaspy, J. A., & Purc-Stephenson, R. (2009). Reporting practice in confirmatory factor analysis: An overview and some recommendations. *Psychological Methods, 14*, 6–23.

Jackson, J. B., Miller, R. B., Oka, M., & Henry, R. G. (2014). Gender differences in marital satisfaction: A meta-analysis. *Journal of Marriage and Family, 76*, 105–129.

Jamieson, L. (1998). *Intimacy: Personal relationships in modern societies*. Cambridge, England: Polity Press.

Karney, B. R., & Bradbury, T. N. (1997). Neuroticism, marital inter-action, and the trajectory of marital satisfaction. *Journal of Personality and Social Psychology, 72*, 1075–1092.

Kiecolt-Glaser, J. K., & Newton, T. L. (2001). Marriage and health: His and hers. *Psychological Bulletin, 127*, 472–503.

Kline, R. B. (2011). *Principles and practice of structural equation modeling* (3rd ed.). New York, NY: Guilford Press.

Locke, H. J., & Wallace, K. M. (1959). Short marital-adjustment and prediction tests: Their reliability and validity. *Marriage and Family Living, 21*, 251–255.

Morgan, D. H. J. (1996). *Family connections: An introduction to family studies*. Cambridge, England: Polity Press.

Morgan, D. H. J. (2011). *Rethinking family practices*. Basingstoke, England: Palgrave Macmillan.

Norton, R. (1983). Measuring marital quality: A critical look at the dependent variable. *Journal of Marriage and the Family, 45*, 141–151.

Proulx, C. M., Helms, H. M., & Buehler, C. (2007). Marital quality and personal well-being: A meta-analysis. *Journal of Marriage and Family, 69*, 576–593.

Sabatelli, R. M. (1988). Measurement issues in marital research: A review and critique of contemporary survey instruments. *Journal of Marriage and the Family, 4*, 891–915.

Schumm, W. R., Nichols, C. W., Schectman, K. L., & Grigsby, C. C. (1983). Characteristics of responses to the Kansas marital satisfaction scale by a sample of 84 married mothers. *Psychological Reports, 53*, 567–572.

Smart, C. (2007). *Personal life*. Cambridge, England: Polity Press.

Spanier, G. B. (1976). Measuring dyadic adjustment: New scales for assessing the quality of marriage and similar dyads. *Journal of Marriage and the Family, 38*, 15–28.

Twenge, J. M., Campbell, W. K., & Foster, C. A. (2003). Parenthood and marital satisfaction: A meta-analytic review. *Journal of Marriage and Family, 65*, 574–583.

Vaughn, M. J., & Baier, M. E. M. (1999). Reliability and validity of the relationship assessment scale. *The American Journal of Family Therapy, 27*, 137–147.

Walker, J., Barrett, H., Wilson, G., & Chang, Y. S. (2010). *Understanding the needs of adults (particularly parents) regarding relationship support* (Research brief DCSF-RBX-10-01). London, England: DCFS.

Walker, R. B., & Luszcz, M. A. (2009). The health and relationship dynamics of late-life couples: A systematic review of the literature. *Ageing and Society, 29*, 455–480.

9 Bisexuality and ageing

Why it matters for social work practice

Kathryn Almack, Rebecca L. Jones and Rachael M. Scicluna

Introduction

In relation to the commonly-used sexual identity labels 'gay', 'lesbian' and 'bisexual', bisexual is often the most invisible category. This invisibility and lack of recognition of the needs of bisexuals across the life course is important to address in the practice of social workers. Taking a life course approach, bisexuality is particularly illustrative of the complex and changing relationships between sexuality and sexual identities. As we shall discuss, it can also make bisexual identities across the life course more visible even if people don't use the identity label of bisexual. Social work has a key role to play in tackling inequalities and their impact in people's lives. In this chapter, we highlight why bisexuality is an urgent matter for social workers to engage with and outline recent empirical evidence that bisexual people are at higher risk of poverty and poor mental health across the life course than lesbians and gay men (Fredriksen-Goldsen, Shiu et al. 2017). This chapter begins with a brief discussion of existing theoretical perspectives on bisexuality. We then introduce empirical research focusing on the lives of bisexual people (albeit it is sparse in contrast to bodies of empirical work addressing the lives of lesbians and gay men). In particular, we focus on what is known about the life course effects of bisexuality and finally we outline the implications for social work practice.

There is scant empirical work related to bisexual people, especially older bisexual people, and what exists comes mainly from the US. This is a gap that our UK study sought to address (Jones, Almack et al. 2016). Finally, we present a discussion of selected case studies from our research to further examine and illustrate key issues in applying research into practice for social workers. Our case studies illustrate ways in which an accumulation of a lifetime of experiences of bisexual people or bisexual relationship histories can lead to what (the editors of this book) identify as 'institutionalized harms', which may be individual, organisational and structural. In turn, there are profound impacts and implications on individual requirements for support, perceptions of support available from social work services, as well as concerns in approaching services, possibly due to past discriminatory experiences for bisexual people.

Theoretical perspectives on bisexuality

Bell (1994) describes bisexuality as very much a place on the margins within LGBT landscapes, acknowledging a fraught relationship between bisexual and gay people, perhaps particularly between bisexual women and lesbians in the context of feminism (Rust 1995). Jones (2010) has also written about the erasure of both bisexual sexualities and sexual identities – when same sex relationships are labelled as lesbian or gay and opposite sex relationships are labelled as heterosexual.

Bisexuality – as sexual orientation *per se* – has been theorised in different ways. This can have implications for social work practice in terms of what is meant or understood when talking about bisexuality. For a more detailed discussion on theoretical perspectives of bisexuality see, for example, Rodriguez-Rust (2000) and Bowes-Catton (2007). One theory set out by Klein (1993) can be particularly useful from a life course perspective. Klein developed a Sexual Orientation Grid, which incorporates seven aspects of sexual identity. While this errs towards putting people into categories which obscures the fluidity of sexuality, it is useful in that it allows for past, present and ideal aspects of sexual identity, and acknowledges that sexuality is highly complex. As Jones (2010:45) observes, this approach 'complicates the question of what makes up a person's sexual identity', including an individual's self-identity but also encompassing behaviours and desires – relating to the ways in which individuals live out their sexual, intimate and/or emotional desires. This acknowledges that people's sexual identities may shift over the life course such that one's identity at one point in time may differ from one's lived experience and identity over one's life course.

Jones (forthcoming) observes how questions about sexual identity can privilege an individual's current sexual identity over any alternative sexual identities they might have claimed in their past. Including a temporal element – asking about both past and current identities – could facilitate more sensitive demographic data collection on a client group. For example, in our *Looking Both Ways* study we asked for information on both past and current sexual identities. This facilitates a life course perspective which can also help make bisexual sexuality and identities more visible too. If the focus is solely on an individual's current sexual identity – or it is assumed on the basis of a current relationship and the gender of the individual's partner – binary assumptions can come into play. Both gender and sexuality are fluid as we shall outline later in our case studies. Other aspects of diversity are important to keep in mind too, recognising intersections between sexual identities with other identities. Intersectionality draws attention to the multiple social positions an individual may occupy simultaneously. As Fish and Karban (2015:5) note:

> Race, disability, class, gender have an impact on people's experiences of discrimination and access to social capital, that is, the personal and collective resources that improve one's educational, economic and social position...

Although the intersectional approach has not been used widely in social work, it offers a useful perspective and its theoretical underpinnings are informed by social justice.

The intersectional approach offers a nuanced perspective of people's lives and can alert social workers to the social injustice that some bisexuals' lives are underpinned with. In the following section, we turn to examine such injustice in more depth.

Life course effects of bisexuality and the implications for social work

As noted, there is little empirical work on the lives of bisexual people, especially older cohorts. A recent US study (Fredriksen-Goldsen, Shiu et al. 2017) gathered a subsample of 174 participants who identified as bisexual (out of a total of 2,560 LGBT participants). Participants had a mean age of 66.7 and overall 13.2% were people of colour. The study tested and confirmed a number of hypotheses – namely that bisexual people would:

- Have poorer health than lesbians and gay men of a similar age
- Be more likely to experience sexual identity disadvantage – lower levels of identity disclosure and elevated internalised stigma combined with lower social resources (for example less sense of belonging to LGBT communities and lower levels of social support compared to lesbians and gay men of similar age)
- Have lower socio-economic status, compared to lesbians and gay men of similar age

The authors stated that:

> … our findings support the idea that the accumulation of disadvantage results in persistent health inequities for bisexuals in older age. The historical context of invisibility and rejection of bisexuality may limit access to resources across the life course, resulting by older age in more limited accumulation of wealth and health that supports optimal aging.
> (2017:475)

These findings are highly relevant for social workers to address; persistent health inequalities and the potential of reduced resources to draw upon may mean that bisexual people are more in need of support from social services. This may be compounded as bisexual adults age. Compared with lesbian and gay older adults, bisexual older adults experienced greater stigma, less identity disclosure, less social support and less community belonging. These findings indicate that disadvantages in social positions observed in working-age bisexuals also extend into older age. High levels of internalized stigma and identity concealment may be barriers to obtaining important social resources that contribute to health and well-being; for example, bisexual adults' relative lack of acceptance into sexual minority communities may limit their access to support and specialized services within these communities. Furthermore, during the ageing process, older adults' social networks often shrink (Ajrouch, Blandon et al. 2005) and they may become more dependent on other types of support services. Thus, bisexual adults may face dual mutually maintained challenges as they age: high need for social and health resources due to the accumulation of disadvantages over time, along with low access to the communities that may be best positioned to address these elevated needs.

There is even less qualitative research about the lives of older bisexual people than there is quantitative research. Where bisexual people are included in qualitative work, sample numbers are so small that they are often subsumed under the LGBT acronym and included on the basis of same sex relationships. This prompted the development of our small study to focus specifically on bisexuality – which developed out of a seminar series which focused on gaps in our knowledge about the lives of older LGBT people.[1] The lives of older lesbians and gay men are gaining more visibility with time. More research is appearing in this field (Pugh 2005; Hughes 2008; Ward, Pugh et al. 2010; Westwood, King et al. 2015; Scicluna 2017), although more needs to be done to raise awareness through training provisions for social workers. However, bisexual people, like transgender people, remain rather hidden in research and care policy (Jones, Almack et al. 2016; Marshall 2017).

Looking Both Ways

Looking Both Ways was a research project exploring the experiences of older bisexual people or people who had had significant bisexual relationships across their lives. We recruited twelve people aged 50 and over who claimed a bisexual identity or who acknowledged a relationship history across their life course which could be seen as bisexual, even if they did not use the label 'bisexual'. The lower-age limit of 50 was adopted in common with most studies of LGBT ageing. Participants were aged 51–83; the majority were in their 50s and 60s and the mean age was 64.

We recruited initially via people who attended a seminar mentioned earlier (see endnote 1) which was addressing the gaps in knowledge about bisexual ageing and extended recruitment using our own networks. We recognised that we could not achieve a representative sample of respondents. Estimating the size and demographic trends of the ageing LGB population is not possible given that there are no official UK demographic statistics on LGB individuals of any age group. Furthermore, sexual orientation does not map neatly on to the sexual identities that people claim, and sexual behaviours do not always map onto sexual identities.

Each participant was interviewed once and interviews lasted between 45 minutes and 3 hours. The interview schedule started with a narrative life history (Wengraf 2001) and then moved to a discussion of issues to do with ageing. With permission, interviews were audio-recorded and transcribed. Emerging themes were identified through individual readings of selected transcripts by the three authors. This thematic analysis continued through further readings and team discussions of the dataset. A coding framework of fifteen nodes was developed and applied to all transcripts, using NVivo software. We then developed summary case studies addressing issues of sexual identity across the life course and about ageing. The case study for each participant was written by the team member who carried out that participant's interview and sent back to the interviewee to check and agree.

The study was granted ethical approval by The Open University's Human Research Ethics Committee and followed the research ethics guidance of the British Society of Gerontology. We acknowledge that the small sample size means that the findings can only be indicative and suggestive. Relating the findings to the existing literature on LGBT ageing more generally, and to Fredriksen-Goldsen and colleagues' quantitative study (Fredriksen-Goldsen, Shiu et al. 2017), makes it possible to make some recommendations based on the diversity found within this small dataset. The next section introduces some of our case studies and offers recommendations for social work practice.

A note on our case studies

We don't know enough about the characteristics of older people with bisexual histories to know what a typical life story would look like. The three case studies presented here may be quite untypical because our sample is small – certainly they have characteristics which are quite uncommon in the wider population, such as having consensually non-monogamous relationships. Although many bisexual people are monogamous, some evidence suggests that some bisexual communities, including the ones to which Ian and Megan are connected, have higher rates of transgender and consensually non-monogamous people in them than the general population (Barker, Bowes-Catton et al. 2008). Our recruitment methods may have led us to an over-representation of individuals within such communities and reflect this rather than being a representative finding about bisexual older people *per se* in the UK.

Case studies from Looking Both Ways

Ian

Ian is 51 and can't recall ever identifying as heterosexual. From an early age he felt attracted to both boys and girls and this continued into adult life, although at the current point in his life he feels more attracted to women than to men. He has lived long-term with a female partner with whom he had a commitment ceremony. They have had a child together. He and his partner are non-monogamous and Ian has always been involved in bisexual communities and continues to be so. Bisexuality has been a consistent identity for Ian throughout his life. Much of the time however, living with a female partner and their child, Ian describes being seen as:

> … utterly heterosexual'. Absolutely. And for me, there is the bi community and there is the rest of my life with a disconnect to an extent between the two of them. I don't bother coming out unless there is a relevant discussion or whatever. I just can't be bothered …
> I am still bisexual there but not necessarily outwardly or vocally.

Ian says he cannot imagine his sexual identity changing as he grows older. He attends a major UK annual event for bisexuals (BiCon) which he describes as a 'lovely space' which has been 'life-changing' for him. He has only ever missed one event. He commented that he has been attending this event for longer than many of the other delegates have been alive which makes him conscious of his age. At the same time, he thinks visible older bisexual role models are important. He reflects that if he needed help with mobility, he would want a carer to be 'OK' with facilitating him going to events like BiCon. In old age, this could be vitally important as a means of mitigating the potential for social isolation from key community resources that enhance Ian's well-being.

The death of his father has made him think more about ageing and later life. Visiting his father in a care home, he was struck by the lack of internet access for residents. This would be important to him:

> I am utterly sure my parents' generation would have been most upset if they didn't have face to face social time with people … and I don't need that. That would come second to having decent internet access, uncensored internet access rather than through a nanny filter. I don't want anyone going why are you looking at this LGB site sort of stuff or anything sexual has been erased … by filters.

He's not sure if he would want to come out as bisexual to carers if cared for at home, especially if they were only coming in briefly or he rarely saw the same person twice. If it was a more full-time relationship with a series of staff, he thinks he might feel more motivated to be open about his sexual identity. Other factors he identified included whether or not he was in a relationship with someone of the same sex who wanted to visit him. Invisibility annoys him in other settings and he feels he might have to make it clear he is not gay but bisexual.

Lack of visibility and potentially fewer opportunities to access affirmative social support can heighten risks to the well-being of older bisexual

people as discussed earlier. Pilkey et al. (Pilkey, Scicluna et al. 2017) identified that having a carer who is blind to sexuality and gender at home can
create anxiety and stress. Much of existing guidance and research about
LGBT ageing fails to pay significant attention to bisexuality, or conflates
bisexual men's experiences with those of gay men, or bisexual women's experiences with those of lesbians (Dworkin 2006). Some of Ian's concerns relate
to this, in relation to being invisible. He identifies aspects of support that
could be incredibly important to him as a bisexual person and as he ages.
For example, how he hopes for support, if needed, to be able to continue
to access bisexual spaces that he finds affirmative. This includes important
social networks but also virtual networks. Ian identifies envisaging sexuality
continuing to be important and raises a valid point about uncensored access
to the Internet. These are all issues that social workers may need to engage
with, including recognition of older people's sexuality and developing understandings of the complex ways sexual identities are expressed.

Megan

Megan, 60, identifies as bisexual and she is in a polyamorous relationship.
She recalls feeling attracted to other women at University although this is
also where she met her then-male partner who she married and had children with. Later in life, the man Megan married transitioned to become a
woman. It was a challenging time for Megan and their relationship, but they
only divorced in order to become civil partners, later converting this to marriage after the passage of the Marriage (Same Sex Couples) Act. Together
they discovered polyamorous and bisexual communities, which gave them
a helpful framework to reconfigure their relationship. They now live with
Paul who became a partner of both of them, and the three of them own the
house they live in together. They all have secondary partners as well. Megan
acknowledges that they are a fairly 'unusual' type of family. She thinks being polyamorous may have benefits in later life, reflecting on a period of time
when she was having treatment for cancer:

> … (my) two partners had each other for support, and they had their
> secondary partners for support, and then they were still able to sup-
> port me, and everything I think was so much smoother because of being
> poly. There was so many more people around to support, and it really
> yeah, we got through that. I think, I know that people when there's just
> two people and there's a cancer diagnosis, it can fracture things so badly
> that you never get it back. And I was so pleased that we had more than
> that. I always think in terms of a relationship with two people. It's kind
> of like a ladder. If it hadn't got something secure to lean on, it's going
> to fall over. If you've got three or more, it's more like a little stool, it's
> stable; it's got three points to stand on.

The above quote brings out a lifestyle and home setting which falls out of the normative domestic setting. However, at the same time, if social workers are unware of 'alternative domesticities' (Pilkey, Scicluna et al. 2015), this may pose difficulties and unnecessary stress to those that are receiving the care, risking prejudice, biphobia and polyphobia. Megan referred to a period of time during treatment when she had surgery. While she convalesced at home, she had a bed set up in a separate room. This was a temporary arrangement and she missed being in the main bedroom with her partners. She felt this shift was difficult to explain to carers coming into the home:

> It was difficult to explain to anybody coming in why this was a change. They would come in, they would see me in that single bed in that single room ... even if they accepted that we are three, they would see they had the main bedroom, and I don't think they would realise or understand that actually normally I would have been in there too, and I would be missing it.

Being outside normative frameworks, it is also possible that individuals within non-traditional relationships may be excluded in a number of ways, if not fully acknowledged. For example, not being able to have an active role in the care of a partner or, after death, by not having their grief acknowledged (Almack, Seymour et al. 2010). It emphasises the importance not to make assumptions about someone's relationships. Megan and her partners may also need support later in life as pensions and financial provision are areas of concern for them, especially for Paul who at the moment has no rights to survivors' benefits from his two partners' pensions.

Chryssy

Chryssy is 52 and identifies as pansexual, with previous sexual identities at different points in time being gay, lesbian and bisexual. Chryssy prefers to use the pronoun 'they' rather than 'she'. Their gender identity is on a 'trans feminine spectrum' and they try to avoid binary categories. In their life, they first identified as gay, which seems a way of explaining why they felt different from their peers. However, being part of a gay scene, Chryysy still felt different and they began to identify quite strongly as bisexual. Chryssy married in their mid-20s and had two children, they also have a daughter from a previous relationship. They were later divorced and moved abroad. Chryssy says:

> I was searching for something that you don't know what is it, but you're searching in areas where you're likely to find these kind of things.

Chryssy's contact with their children was disrupted, although they now has a good relationship with the children from their marriage and is rebuilding a relationship with their daughter. They have been in and out of relationships but they are more interested in:

> ... establishing actual community across people with these by now established non-normative identities.

They live in a shared rented flat. Chryssy would describe themselves as 'materially poor' and to a large extent that ties in with the way they have led their life. One of the consequences of the life they had led, searching for who they were and making sense of their gendered and sexual identities, is that they have moved around a lot and spent periods of time abroad. That can disrupt opportunities to build up resources – such as pension funds, owning one's own home, a secure income and employment rights that increase over time in a job. This can have consequences for an individual's future. Chryssy volunteers for a project working with older people and does wonder about their future. They envisage developing a 'like-minded' community:

> ... some kind of communal living, which could be flats or could be a neighbourhood or some housing composite in London around neighbourhoods. And with likeminded people, not similar, not everyone the same but with likeminded people. But with an ethos that is, it's to do with sharing. I'm a hopeless gardener, I'm not interested really, but sharing gardens. In payment for people doing my garden I'll do their washing up, that's absolutely fine. Those kind of approaches. So we're not talking there about the intimacy of living, we're talking about the practicality of living and support on hand.

It is important to take into account the ways in which an accumulation of a lifetime of experiences of bisexual people or bisexual relationship histories can impact on one's life. These life histories may have cumulative and profound impacts on an individual in terms of their mental and physical health as well as material resources they have access to, social support and so on. In part, these issues can be attributed to 'minority stress', a conceptual framework developed by Meyer (Meyer 2003, 2007). Minority stress encompasses experiences of stigma, marginalisation or discrimination, which may have a significant bearing on the health and well-being of LGB people (Mulé, Ross et al. 2009, GLMA (Gay and Lesbian Medical Association) 2010). Bisexuals in older age can face an accumulation of disadvantage which in turn results in persistent and greater health inequities for bisexuals than for lesbians and gay men. As noted earlier, there is increasing evidence that bisexual people are at higher risk of poverty and poor mental health across the life course than lesbians and gay men (Fredriksen-Goldsen, Shiu et al. 2017). Bisexual experiences are often collapsed into lesbian and gay issues, contributing to the invisibility that the bisexual community contends with and bisexual people face dual discrimination and invisibility within heteronormative and lesbian/gay spaces.

Social workers aim 'to promote social justice and social change with and on behalf of clients and the communities in which they live and circumstances in which they exist' (Bailey 2015:xxiii). They are positioned well to mitigate and prevent problems that may arise as a result of the minority stress that bisexual people face in their lifetime. At the same time, it is important to note that sexual minorities can also display considerable resilience and strategies to thrive – often through the development of supportive and affirmative networks of 'like-minded' people. Health and social support is often instigated – through policy and practice – from a premise of focusing primarily on family (hetero)relationships, with a particular emphasis on support and care giving biased towards families constructed by marriage or blood ties (Manthorpe 2003). It is important to take account of other important social relationships. Young, Seale, et al. (1998) note, for example, the wider neglect of the role of friendship and informal social networks.

Bisexual people and people with a life course history which may seem bisexual even if they don't identify as bisexual will be users of social work services. Thus, our findings speak to social work's mandate of embracing diversity. Social workers support people at critical times in their lives and it is important to address bisexuality even if it is a sexual identity label that some may reject or find constraining for a number of reasons.

Applying research findings to professional practice

Bisexuality matters because

- There is evidence of higher levels of mental and physical health problems for bisexual people attributed to minority stress
- They are at risk of poorer quality care because providers do not always understand or fully consider their needs
- Their relationships and support networks are not always immediately recognisable within normative frameworks
- People who don't identify as bisexual may still have a history of relationships with more than one gender – this means care should be taken not to make assumptions about who are the significant people in their life
- People may identify as bisexual when they are single or in a monogamous same-sex or different-sex couple relationship. Bisexuality encompasses sexual behaviour but also attractions, desires and identity
- There are limited safe spaces to express a bisexual identity or interests – including within care settings or receiving care at home

- There may be negative perceptions of support available from social work services, as well as concerns in approaching services possibly due to past discriminatory experiences
- People may identify as bisexual when they are single or in a monogamous same-sex or different-sex couple relationship
- The importance of addressing bisexuality in relation to class, age, wealth, ethnicity and so on.

Questions and issues for social workers to reflect upon

- How might a social worker explore and identify important aspects of someone's sexuality and sexual identity – without falling back on heteronormative assumptions
- What might be the most appropriate ways to work with a client's network of support in a sensitive manner
- There is a need for honest reflexive practice through training – self-awareness and checking assumptions don't inadvertently creep in. Not all clients may feel safe in 'coming out' about a bisexual life-course or identity. How might social workers approach such reflexivity?

Note

1 The seminar was one of six in a seminar series funded by the Economic and Social Research Council entitled *Older Lesbian, Gay, Bisexual and Trans People: Minding the Knowledge Gaps* (King, A., Almack. K., Suen, Y.T. and Westwood, S.) www.surrey.ac.uk/sociology/research/researchcentres/crag/seminar_series/.

References

Ajrouch, K. J., A. Y. Blandon, T. C. Antonucci (2005). Social networks among men and women: The effects of age and socioeconomic status. *The Journals of Gerontology: Series B* 60 (6), S311–S317.
Almack, K., J. Seymour, G. Bellamy (2010). Exploring the impact of sexual orientation on experiences and concerns about end of life care and on bereavement for lesbian, gay and bisexual elders. *Sociology* 44(5), 908–924.
Bailey, G. (2015). Foreword. In: *Lesbian, Gay, Bisexual and Trans Health Inequalities: International Persepectives in Social Work*. J. Fish and K. Karban (eds.), Bristol: Policy Press, xxi–xxv.
Barker, M., H. Bowes-Catton, A. Iantaffi, A. Cassidy, L. Brewer (2008). British bisexuality: A snapshot of bisexual identities in the UK. *Journal of Bisexuality* 8 (1–2) 141–162.
Bell, D. (1994). Bisexuality: A place on the margins. In: *The Margins of the City: Gay Men's Urban Lives*. S. Whittle (ed.), Aldershot: Arena, 129–141.
Bowes-Catton, H. (2007). Resisting the binary: Discourses of identity and diversity in bisexual politics 1988–1996. *Lesbian and Gay Psychology Review* 8 (1), 58–70.

Dworkin, S. H. (2006). Aging bisexual: The invisible of the invisble minority. In: *Lesbian, Gay, Bisexual and Transgender Aging: Research and Clinical Perspectives.* D. Kimmel, T. Rose and S. David (eds.), New York: Columbia University Press.

Fish, J., K. Karban (2015). *Lesbian, Gay, Bisexual and Trans Health Inequalities: International Perspectives in Social Work.* Bristol: Policy Press.

Fredriksen-Goldsen, K. I., C. Shiu, A. E. B. Bryan, J. Goldsen, H.-J. Kim (2017). Health equity and aging of bisexual older adults: Pathways of risk and resilience. *The Journals of Gerontology: Series B* 72 (3), 468–478.

GLMA (Gay and Lesbian Medical Association) (2010). *Healthy People 2010: A Companion Document for LGBT Health.* San Francisco: GLMA.

Hughes, M. (2008). Imagined futures and communities: Older lesbian and gay people's narratives on health and aged care. *Journal of Gay & Lesbian Social Services* 20 (1–2), 167–186.

Jones, R. L. (2010). Troubles with bisexuality in health and social care. In: *LGBT Issues: Looking Beyond Categories.* R. L. Jones and R. Ward (eds.), Edinburgh: Dunedin Academic Press, 42–55.

Jones, R. L., K. Almack, R. M. Scicluna (2016). *Ageing and Bisexuality: Case Studies from the 'Looking Both Ways' Project.* Milton Keynes: Open University.

Klein, F. (1993). *The Bisexual Option.* New York: Haworth Press.

Manthorpe, J. (2003). Nearest and dearest? The neglect of lesbians in caring relationships. *British Journal of Social Work* 33 (6), 753–768.

Marshall, L. (2017). Castle and cell: Exploring intersections between sexuality and gender in the domestic lives of men with trans identities and histories. In: *Gender and Sexuality at Home: Experience, Politics, Transgression.* B. Pilkey, R. M. Scicluna and B. Campkin (eds.), London: Bloomsbury.

Meyer, I. H. (2003). Prejudice, social stress, and mental health in lesbian, gay, and bisexual populations: Conceptual issues and research evidence. *Psychological Bulletin* 129 (5), 674–697.

Meyer, I. (2007). Prejudice and discrimination as social stressors. In: *The Health of Sexual Minorities.* I. Meyer (ed.), New York: Springer.

Mulé, N. J., L. E. Ross, B. Deeprose, B. E. Jackson, A. Daley, A. Travers, D. Moore (2009). Promoting LGBT health and wellbeing through inclusive policy development. *International Journal for Equity in Health* 8 (1), 18.

Pilkey, B., R. M. Scicluna, A. Gorman-Murray (2015). Alternative domesticities. *Home Cultures* 12 (2), 127–138.

Pilkey, B., R. M. Scicluna, B. Campkin, B. Penner (2017). *Gender and Sexuality at Home: Experience, Politics, Transgression.* London: Bloomsbury.

Pugh, S. (2005). Assessing the cultural needs of older lesbians and gay men: Implications for practice. *Practice (UK)* 17 (3), 207–218.

Rodriguez-Rust, P. (2000). *Bisexuality in the United States: A Social Science Reader.* New York: Columbia University Press.

Rust, P. (1995). *Bisexuality and the Challenge to Lesbian Politics: Sex, Loyalty, and Revolution.* New York and London: New York University Press.

Scicluna, R. M. (2017). *Home and Sexuality: The 'Other' Side of the Kitchen.* London: Palgrave Macmillan.

Ward, R., S. Pugh, E. Price (2010). *Don't Look Back? Improving Health and Social Care Service Delivery for Older LGB Users.* London: Equality and Human Rights Commission.

Wengraf, T. (2001). *Qualitative Research Interviewing: Biographic Narrative and Semi-Structured Methods.* London: Sage.

Westwood, S., A. King, K. Almack, Y. T. Suen, L. Bailey (2015). Good practice in health and social care provision for LGBT older people in the UK. In: *Lesbian, Gay, Bisexual and Trans Health Inequalities: International Persepctives in Social Work.* J. Fish and K. Karban (eds.), Bristol: Policy Press.

Young, E., C. Seale, M. Bury (1998). 'It's not like family going is it?': Negotiating friendship boundaries towards the end of life. *Mortality: Promoting the Interdisciplinary Study of Death and Dying* 3 (1), 27–42.

10 Single women living alone in later life

Evidence from Understanding Society data

Hafiz T.A. Khan, Trish Hafford-Letchfield and Nicky Lambert

Introduction

This chapter picks up the study of gender issues within ageing populations. According to OECD statistics, the UK is the loneliest country in Europe and the least likely to report having close friendships or knowing their neighbours (OECD, 2005). The number of people living on their own has doubled since the 1970s, with single-person households now making up a third of all homes. We report on the findings of our examination of some of the factors associated with health and well-being of women living alone in later life using data collected in the 'Understanding Society' 2012. This is a nationwide longitudinal survey that captures important information on the life course trajectories of individuals in the UK. By looking at variables associated with health and well-being, we have identified some relevant determinants when looking at single older women living alone. The prevalence of living alone during later life varies widely across developed countries, but everywhere its growth has been remarkable in recent decades, even in societies with traditionally strong family ties (Reher and Requena, 2017). Within the increasing trend of single women living alone over time and space, there is a need to adapt and develop more accurate measures and research designs in order to begin to understand the factors impacting on the nature of ageing for those who are living alone. Forming new intimate relationships might be one way of compensating for any loneliness associated with this phenomenon (Carr, 2004).

Gender issues in ageing researchAs we will see in the following chapter, the importance of comparing profiles for different groups of older women is useful to consider the development of research priorities which support inclusive positive ageing. Household status and living arrangements are important for individuals to satisfy several goals (Burch and Matthews, 1987), for example, privacy, companionship and care, and socio-psychological costs such as staying connected as well as for practical reasons as in making domestic arrangements and economies of scale. Chapter 11 considers further how these are often impacted upon by opportunities in earlier life associated with relationships and fertility. Reher and Requena (2017) also refer to macro-, meso- and micro-level contexts (see also Dykstra, 2009), and living alone has been shown to be directly linked to higher levels of disease and disability (Kharicha et al., 2007). For those of us working in care services, we need to be aware of the potential for how living alone lowers the levels of social and familial support in later life (Hafford-Letchfield et al., 2016), and not only the risk of having insufficient support but the potential loss of quality in relationships including sexuality and intimacy.

This chapter picks up the study of gender issues within ageing populations now of global interest given that women represent just under half of the population (Powell and Khan, 2013). Understanding different life trajectories and diversity characteristics of the ageing female population is important given the implications for wider society and culture. Women's changing circumstances, attitudes and behaviours are affecting their experience of ageing at both an individual and societal level. These circumstances present new opportunities and challenges for governments, policy-makers and service providers. As life expectancy increases, the 'traditional' life-stage trajectory is changing (Laslett, 1994; Kirkwood, 2014). The 2015 World Population Prospects (UN, 2015) confirms that significant gains in life expectancy have been achieved worldwide. During 2010–2015, global average life expectancy was estimated to be 70.48 years, which is predicted to be 79.18 years by 2060–2065. On the contrary, in more developed regions, life expectancy was 78.30 years during 2010–2015 and this will increase to 85.38 by 2060–2065. In the UK, life expectancy at birth for males and females are 78.45 and 82.39 years respectively during 2010–2015 with evidence of increasing longevity in later life (ONS, 2014a; UN, 2015). Centenarians are increasing at a faster rate than any other age group too; an over 137-fold increase between 1911 and 2013 (from 100 to 13,780) (ONS, 2014b).

Changes to the life course, life stages and lifestyle choices are starting to have a marked impact on the shape, size and types of households in the UK (Laslett, 1994; McNair, 2009) as well as the biographies of current generations of older people (Bildtgard and Oberg, 2017). Single women living alone may reflect a lifestyle choice as well as the consequences of other influencing factors, such as loss of a partner through separation, divorce or death (Victor et al, 2000; Hafford-Letchfield et al., 2016). More than three and a half million people in the UK aged 65+ live alone, which corresponds to 32 percent of all people aged 65+ in the UK, of which nearly 70 percent are women (ONS, 2016). Out of the 2 million people over 75 who live alone, 1.5 million of these are also women (ONS, 2016). Further, 61 percent of widows (male and female) in England and Wales are aged 75 and over. Living alone may be a result of the inability to find the right relationship at the right time as well the use of fertility control or the experience of fertility problems in earlier life (Al-Kandari and Crews, 2014). Besides these more commonly perceived reasons for living alone in later life, greater diversity in relationship status has also been influenced by choice and sexual identities, for example, evidence suggests that older lesbian, gay, bisexual and transgender people are more likely to live alone in old age, with fewer links with younger generations, thereby increasing their risk of isolation (Heaphy and Yip, 2003). Within this group, older lesbians are likely to live longer than (gay) men, to be less well off in later life and to make greater use of health and social care services (Trais, 2016). Further, studies of non-familial relationships – 'families of choice' (Weeks et al., 2001) or 'friendship families' (Dorfman et al., 1995) – and those roles of caregivers and care receivers may be fluid, interchangeable and context-dependent. In the absence of positive and powerful counter narratives, the notion of living alone by choice or circumstances is a powerful and uncontested one with less interrogation into these different identities. Against this background, academic research on 'living alone' in later life is one area that is relatively underdeveloped in relation to its different causes, manifestations and explanations.

Living alones in British households

Within British households, this study shows that over the last three to four decades, there has been a considerable increase in the number of people living alone (Pampel, 1992; Legare and Martel, 2003; Macvarish, 2006). Demographers have identified that this trajectory starts to emerge during midlife and have observed increasing trends among men living alone in the UK (Demey et al., 2011, 2013). Some studies have shown that older women living alone are more likely to possess relatively less material resources than their male counterparts (Eurostat, 2002; Gaymu and Springer, 2010), and in many cases are dependent on their children and relatives (Khan and Leeson, 2006). Longer life is also associated with multiple morbidities and long-term care. Whilst many enjoy longer longevity compared to the previous generation, they also need to prepare for supporting themselves in circumstances which may also coexist with increasing social isolation (Banks et al., 2009) and lack of both economic and practical support, particularly where there is a burden of care (Maynard et al., 2008; Laing and Buisson, 2014). Women living alone may not be able to draw on the range of family and community support often seen in many societies (Lee and Xiao, 1998; Kohli, 1999; Khan, 2014; Hafford-Letchfield et al., 2016). As mentioned earlier, some studies are beginning to pick up these issues much earlier (Demey et al., 2013) which is important given that UK legislation and policy on care entitlement and provision tends to be underpinned by assumptions about informal care. These assume that all older people will have carers to support them drawn from their family and networks (Hafford-Letchfield, 2013). These expectations may be compromised for single women living alone in later life, as well as for those who have lost a partner. Both groups may have restricted support networks to rely or fall back upon (Kalogirou and Murphy 2006; Girling and Morgan, 2014; DEMOS, 2014).

The attention on women living alone in ageing studies has emerged from disciplines such as sociology, psychology, gender and sexuality studies (Wolf, 1995; Byrne, 2008; Lahad and Hazan, 2014; Girling and Morgan, 2014; Timonen and Doyle, 2014). The aim of this chapter is to review one particular source of demographic data alongside this literature to review any research possibilities which would facilitate better examination of possible trajectories of single older women living alone in British households.

Rationale for the variables selected

We know that the defining characteristics of the ageing process make individuals more vulnerable to disease, disability and frailty, and that in developed nations, the majority of health resources are focused on conditions where age is the biggest risk factor (Kirkwood, 2014). Education has also been associated with socio-economic status, which in turn impacts on health inequalities in later life (McNair, 2009; Rahman et al., 2016). The World Health Organisation defines health as 'a complete physical, mental and social-wellbeing and not merely the absence of disease or infirmity' (2006, p. 5), thus placing emphasis on well-being which goes beyond the existence of physical health. Subjective well-being involves an overall assessment of how people are doing without being directive about what particular aspects of their lives contribute towards their feelings of well-being (Gaymu and Sringer, 2010). However, well-being can be measured in a wide variety of ways. In this paper, we have utilised the variable of 'general happiness' as an indicator of the overall well-being of an individual. Health status is also directly linked with well-being which includes general life satisfaction (Khan and Raeside, 2014, Kirkwood, 2014). Hank and Wagner (2013) have addressed the question of whether and how parenthood and marital status are associated with various dimensions of older peoples' well-being, including elements of the individual's economic situation, psychological well-being and social connectedness. Gaymu and Springer's (2010) European study of the influences of objective living conditions on the life satisfaction of older Europeans living alone from a gender and cross-national perspective, found that a lower proportion of women living alone declared themselves to be satisfied with life compared to men. When controlling for inequalities in living conditions, this difference disappeared. Gamu and Springer found that determinants of older women's life satisfaction, however, were more strongly linked to the sociocultural. Other studies have also found that despite less favourable conditions, older women report only slightly lower life satisfaction, happiness and self-esteem (Pinquart and Sorensen 2001; Inglehart, 2002). These different findings have led to debates about the need for gender specific models to measure well-being (Pinquart and Sorensen 2001; Hafford-Letchfield, 2016). These would take into account institutional differences that influence gender inequalities in the living conditions of older people living alone as well as both objective and subjective measures. An example of such study involved a secondary phenomenological analysis of studies exploring the concept of 'hope' in the everyday life of older women living alone (Porter et al., 2011). Porter et al. (2011) produced a descriptive taxonomy of their life-world pertaining to 'hoping'. This taxonomy found that the woman's preferred futures involved both the mundane and the profound, but were still focused firmly on 'living'.

Methodology

The study uses UK *Understanding Society* data. The data enables us to examine individual behaviour both cross-sectional and through the life course. The data is scientifically rich enough to capture key determinants of health outcomes within UK society. The study is an annual survey of each adult member of a nationally representative sample. The same individuals are re-interviewed in each wave. If individuals leave their household, all adult members of their new household are interviewed. Each wave is collected over 24 months, such that the first wave of data was collected between January 2009 and 2011, the second wave between January 2010 and 2012, and so forth. Each person aged 16 or older answers the individual adult interview and self-completion questionnaire. Young people aged 10–15 years are asked to respond to a paper self-completion questionnaire (UK data service, 2015). As definition and their measurements are available in the main documents of understanding society manual (McFall, 2013) we have not gone into further detail here.

The target population for analysis in this paper are women who were defined as being aged 55 years plus and living alone in the household. In the survey, a question was asked about number of own children in the household (specific survey code c_nchild_dv) that includes natural children, adopted children and step children under age of 16 years. The survey Understanding Society uses a single_dv code to enumerate those living alone in the household. This target group of sample was then subject to detailed data analysis. Both exogenous as well as endogenous variables were used for model building purposes in this paper. Exogenous variables are free dependency in the model whereas endogenous are those which are used at least once as a dependent variable in the model building stages. Thus five exogenous variables are used in Figure 10.1 (age, belong(ing) to a social website, sexual orientation, highest qualification and place of residence) and four endogenous variables (long-standing illness or disability, health limits modern activities, satisfaction with health, health status and general happiness).

The detailed category of each variable is given in Table 10.1 and these were subsequently used for statistical analysis. The Understanding Society survey questionnaire is made available online for any further consultation or verification.

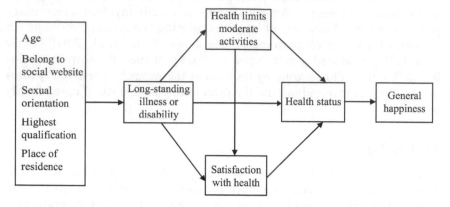

Figure 10.1 Path diagram showing linkages between selected variables considered in the study about here.

Table 10.1 Characteristics of general population as well as study population about here

Characteristics	Total sample		Women 55+ living alone	
	Cases	%	Cases	%
Gender				
Male	22,788	45.8	3,830	7.7
Female	26,951	54.2		
Age				
55–64	7,488	15.1	1,155	30.2
65–74	5,975	12.0	1,157	30.2
75–84	3,246	6.5	421	28.6
85+	848	1.7	389	11.0
Belong to social website				
Yes	20,722	41.7	389	10.5
No	25,159	50.6	3,314	89.5
Sexual orientation				
Heterosexual	38,008	76.4	2,836	93.6
Gay or lesbian	476	1.0	9	0.3
Bisexual	406	0.8	9	0.3
Other	424	0.9	32	1.1
Prefer not to say	1,296	2.6	143	4.7
Highest qualification				
Degree	10,822	21.8	361	9.6
Other higher degree	5,405	10.9	470	12.5
A-level etc.	10,175	20.5	300	8.0
GCSE etc.	10,305	20.7	532	14.1

(Continued)

Characteristics	Total sample		Women 55+ living alone	
	Cases	%	Cases	%
Other qualification	4,769	9.6	590	15.7
No qualification	7,190	14.5	1,509	40.1
Place of residence				
Urban area	37,740	75.9	2850	74.4
Rural area	11,980	24.1	979	25.6
General health				
Excellent	8,760	17.6	300	7.8
Very good	16,956	34.1	934	24.4
Good	13,290	26.7	1,009	26.4
Fair	7,443	15.0	1,020	26.6
Poor	3,247	6.5	566	14.8
Long-standing illness or disability				
Yes	17,130	34.4	2,403	62.8
No	32,561	65.5	1,424	37.2
Health limits moderate activities				
Yes, limited a lot	3,351	8.2	703	23.1
Yes, limited a little	7,252	17.8	885	29.1
No, not limited at all	30,108	74.4	1,455	47.8
General happiness				
More so than usual	4,511	11.1	193	6.4
About the same as usual	30,669	75.4	2,450	80.7
Less so than usual	4,472	11.0	314	10.3
Much less than usual	1,014	2.5	78	2.6
Satisfaction with health				
Completely dissatisfied	2,429	4.9	213	7.0
Mostly dissatisfied	5,557	11.2	445	14.7
Somewhat dissatisfied	5,707	11.5	508	16.7
Neither satisfied or dissatisfied	3,194	6.4	290	9.6
Somewhat satisfied	5,339	10.7	457	15.1
Mostly satisfied	14,488	29.1	927	30.6
Completely satisfied	3,943	7.9	194	6.4

Analytical framework

Descriptive statistics, cross-tabulation and multivariate logistic re-
gressions are used to examine key variables associated with health and
well-being of older women who are living alone. Selected variables are
considered in the paper as to examine how they are interrelated. Variables
are considered as categorical as seen in the list in Table 10.1. A schematic
diagram describes the links and causality between variables for analysis
(see Figure 10.1).

Statistical analyses

Exploratory data analysis (EDA) was carried out to understand the selected characteristics of respondents, mainly the frequency analysis of variables for the selected subcategories. Bivariate analysis was performed to compare the difference between sub-groups of each independent variable and the significance of difference was measured by the Chi-squared tests. Finally, a multivariate logistic regression model was employed to explore the factors affecting health status and general happiness (well-being) among older women living alone while controlling for various predictors. A detailed discussion on logistic regression and its application can be found elsewhere (see for example, Khan and Raeside, 1997; Hosmer and Lemeshow, 2000; Khan, 2014).

Results

The data analysis was performed based on a study population of older women living alone in a British household. Their socio-economic and demographic characteristics were analysed. As women live longer than men, it is anticipated that the proportion of older women living alone will increase as they get older. Three waves of data (Waves 1, 2 and 3) were used to capture a picture of this trend as well as its distribution within the individual population. Table 10.1 shows the percent distribution of men and women in single British households by considering five years age groups. The data reveals that the number of women in single British households is higher than number of men in single British households across these three waves. In wave 1 there were as many as 1,890 men and 3,912 women, in wave 2 (1,665 men and 3,317 women) and in wave 3 (1,939 men and 3,830 women).

A total of 49,739 individuals (males = 22,788 and females = 26,951) were surveyed in wave 3 in which the proportion of women living in single households is estimated to be 7.7 percent. There has been a significant variation in number of women by age cohort and the proportion is found to be higher for upper age groups. For example, in wave 3, only 14.6 percent of women living in single households belong to age group 55–59 years, whereas it is 54.3 percent for age group 70 years or above. This indicates that there are a higher proportion of older women living alone without a partner and any dependents in the household.

The vast majority of women living alone live in England compared with other regions and the sample is well representative of the country's population size. Despite a higher sample in England, in all four geographical regions the most common scenario is that a higher proportion of women living alone are in the age range of 70 years or more. As life expectancy continues to increase, the absolute number or proportion of women living alone is projected to increase further on the basis of familial and social changes as discussed earlier in the introduction. This also indicates that a proportional increase in independent living in British households may be linked to the availability of appropriate social support (Lee and Xiao, 1998; Rahman et al., 2004; Al-Kandari and Crews, 2014; Khan et al., 2015). The provision of intergenerational support is particularly pertinent which has been shown to promote filial obligation and transactional approaches to resource transfer in later life (Silverstein et al., 2012; Khan, 2014) and the need for different models of sustainable health and social care provision (DEMOS, 2014). The issue of intergenerational support has become particularly significant given wider recognition for the 'families of choice' that LGB individuals rely on as opposed to more traditional connections with biological kin (Heaphy and Yip, 2003). Research has shown that older lesbian, gay and bisexual adults are not necessarily in contact with families of birth, are less likely to have children in this cohort and family members may not be involved in future care planning or be available (or requested) to provide unpaid care (Hughes, 2009).

As part of exploratory data analysis, a frequency distribution of total sample as well as single women living alone is presented in Table 10.1. This provided us an opportunity to compare women in the study as compared with the entire dataset. The study shows that single household women represent about 8 percent of the total study sample. As the proportion of single women was greater for those who are 70 years or more, we then further regrouped the age group into 10 years age cohorts (55–64, 65–74, 75–84 and 85+ years) to distribute sample equally and to control the variability within each age cohort. This was justified on the basis that disability tends to be linked in later age groups, say 80 years or more (Kirkwood, 2014). A vast majority (about 89.5 percent) of single women in the survey reported that they do not utilise social websites and 93.6 percent identified themselves as heterosexual. About 40 percent had no formal education followed by 29.8 percent who have been educated up to GCSE and A level. The survey also shows that one quarter of single women living alone live in rural areas (25.6 percent). About 15 percent of these women reported that their health condition is poor, more than double of the total sample (6.5 percent). Similarly, single women living alone in the survey reported higher long-standing illness or disability (62.8 percent), to the extent that health limits doing moderate activities (52.2 percent). Conversely, about 58.6 percent of the women reported that their health situation is at least good or even better. Moderate happiness is found to be lower for women living alone (6.4 percent) than the total population (11.1 percent). The percentage univariate analysis does not say anything about how the individual characteristic is linked with health and well-being in later life.

It may be hypothesised that there is no relationship between an individual health status and other selected characteristics of the individual. We considered five exogenous variables, such as age of individual, whether or not they used a social website, their sexual orientation, educational qualification and place of residence in order to examine their association with long-standing illness or disability and whether health limits moderate activities, satisfaction with health, health status and general happiness. The analysis reveals that age is related with long-standing illness or disability ($p < 0.000$) which implies that there is a higher chance of suffering from long-standing illness or disability as we age. Similarly, age is found to be related with moderate activities, satisfaction with health, health status and general happiness even.

Being able to access and having the opportunity to maintain online social relationships is perhaps important for older people living alone and when done extensively has been demonstrated as one of the key elements of aging well (McNair, 2009; Ballantyne et al., 2010). Sourbati (2004) has explored how internet-based delivery of social healthcare related information and services presents any benefits to older people who use care support. A study by Ofcom identified that in the UK, only 33 percent of adults aged 75 years and over had ever used the Internet. Use of the Internet in later life has been shown to influence people in a variety of ways. This can influence their health and provide a means for developing a reliable and supportive social network that can shape well-being that shapes peoples' lives (Hafford-Letchfield, 2011; Thanakwang and Soonthorndhada, 2011). The sample studied here bears out these findings in that there was a statistical association between belonging to a social network with health status and general happiness.

Whilst sexual orientation was found to be unrelated with any of the health and happiness variables, there is increasing and significant research emerging on the association between sexual orientation, identity, culture and lifestyle in later life with impact on health and well-being. This can be both positive and negative, the latter which is associated with being invisible and experiencing homophobic or transphobic discrimination (Willis et al., 2016). Gabrielson and Holston (2014) suggest that lesbian older women, for example, have triple vulnerability (gender, sexual orientation and age) necessitating inquiry into their social support needs and in their study found that older lesbians without children accessed support from 'families of choice' with whom they shared common values and common passion contributing to their sense of well-being and happiness. More research needs to be done with lesbian, bisexual and transgender women in relation to single lifestyles and happiness within the appropriate cultural context. Given that the survey does not ask about gender identity or detailed questions about sexual orientation, we were not able to undertake any analysis of this important group of women.

The multivariate logistic regression is used to identify important variables as well as to measure the extent to which they influence on the dependent variable while controlling for all other remaining variables. The adjusted coefficient reflects the actual effect of variable in the paper and we use only odds ratio (OR) and their 95 percent confidence intervals (CI). In this chapter, we have five dependent variables in which three being treated as endogenous variable (long-standing illness or disability, health limits moderate activities, satisfaction with health) and two other variables being as ultimate dependent variables (Health status, general happiness or well-being).

Table 10.2 Cross-tabulations between characteristics of older women in the household about here

Characteristics	Long-standing illness or disability (% yes)	Health limits moderate activities (% yes)	Satisfaction with health (% dissatisfied)	Health status (% poor health)	General happiness (% not happy)
Age					
55–64	56.8	42.4	51.2	37.1	18.8
65–74	61.7	45.9	44.1	37.4	11.5
75–84	65.9	62.8	48.4	47.4	8.2
85+	74.1	80.1	48.3	48.7	10.0
Chi-square value	*45.7*	*172.4*	*10.0*	*41.4*	*50.8*
Significance p-level	*.000*	*.000*	*.018*	*.000*	*.000*
Belong to social website					
Yes	59.8	43.2	51.7	31.6	17.5
No	62.5	53.4	47.5	41.2	12.3
Chi-square value	*1.0*	*13.2*	*2.2*	*13.2*	*7.6*
Significance p-level	*.296*	*.000*	*.137*	*.000*	*.006*
Sexual orientation					
Heterosexual	60.7	51.7	48.0	36.9	12.9
Gay, lesbian & others	62.2	58.0	47.2	40.4	12.4
Chi-square value	*0.1*	*2.8*	*0.1*	*0.9*	*0.0*
Significance p-level	*.676*	*.090*	*.814*	*.331*	*.837*
Highest qualification					
Degree	53.0	39.5	40.4	25.2	10.5
A-level etc.	56.7	52.5	47.5	37.0	16.7
GCSE etc.	55.6	44.0	47.6	34.6	14.9
Other qualification	69.1	60.4	51.9	49.9	12.8
Chi-square value	*85.4*	*101.8*	*26.6*	*165.0*	*9.1*
Significance p-level	*.000*	*.000*	*.000*	*.000*	*.028*
Place of residence					
Urban area	63.7	53.1	49.6	43.0	12.8
Rural area	60.3	49.7	43.3	37.0	13.1
Chi-square value	*3.6*	*2.6*	*9.3*	*10.7*	*0.1*
Significance p-level	*.056*	*.103*	*.002*	*.001*	*.842*

Note: Sexual orientation is grouped as heterosexual and others. All higher degree is considered in one category and similarly no qualification and other qualification being considered as a separate group. Satisfaction with health is recoded into two groups as dissatisfied (completely dissatisfied, mostly dissatisfied, somewhat dissatisfied and neither satisfied or dissatisfied) and satisfied (somewhat satisfied, mostly satisfied, and completely satisfied). Health limits moderate activities variable is grouped as yes (limited a lot and yes, limited a little), no (not limited at all). General health is grouped as being poor (fair and poor) and good (excellent, very good and good). General happiness is recoded as a dichotomy variable, not happy (less so than usual and much less than usual) and happy (more so than usual and about the same as usual).

Models are constructed as per the analytical framework in Figure 10.1 and this requires inclusion of variables for the dependent variable. So, considering selected covariates we have constructed Model 1 for long-standing illness or disability. Age was found to have significant influence on long-standing illness or disability and Model I shows that the higher the age the more likely that the person is to have suffered from illness or disability. The result shows that cohort 85 years or more has 2.252 times (95% CI: 1.631–3.110) higher likelihood of reporting a long-standing illness or disability than those in the younger age cohort (55–64 years). This may be explained as an expected finding as mobility chance is higher in old ages. Education is found to play important role too. The higher the education, the lower the chance of suffering from long-standing illness or disability.

Model 2 is constructed to tease out the extent to which the selected variables are associated with health limits moderate activities. It has been revealed that age has positive influence on moderate activities, which means that an older person has a higher chance of limiting moderate activities and it is 4.11 times more likely for 85+ age cohort compare to 55–64 years age cohort. Education is significantly related with limiting moderate activities as well. The result shows that higher education lowers the chance of limiting moderate activities. Long-standing illness or disability is found to be strongly related with limiting moderate activities. As can be seen from Table 10.3 that long-standing illness has 6.798 times higher chance of limiting moderate activities than those are not suffering from long-standing illness. This is statistically significant as indicated by p-value and lower and upper limit of confidence intervals ($p < 0.000$, 95% CI: 5.724–8.073).

Model 3 is considered "satisfaction with health" as dependent variable in two outcomes is present (dissatisfied and satisfied). In other words, this model aims to identify key factors related to dissatisfaction with health. It has been found that age is statistically related with dissatisfaction with health. As we age there is higher chance of dissatisfaction and this is reflected in Table 10.3. The oldest old age group has the biggest chance of having dissatisfaction compare to age cohort 55–64 years. This is an expected result (Scharf et al., 2004).

In this sample, education was found to reduce the level of dissatisfaction in women living alone. Education is demonstrated as an important determinant for health and happiness among this group of women. The benefits of education and learning, particularly programmes and interventions which engage older people are beginning to be increasingly researched (McNair, 2009; Hafford-Letchfield, 2011; Hafford-Letchfield and Lavender, 2015; Hafford-Letchfield, 2016). These have made some clear links between education and well-being, for example, through its significance for cognitive performance, health literacy and an increased level of participation through the process and structures associated with education and learning.

However, in the rural sample, nearly 43 percent of women in our category were reported as having poorer health as compared to 37 percent in the

Table 10.3 Logistic regression result displays the important factors influencing the dependent variables

Covariates	Long-standing illness or disability (% yes) Model 1	Health limits moderate activities (% yes) Model 2	Satisfaction with health (% dissatisfied) Model 3	Health status (% poor health) Model 4	General happiness (% not happy) Model 5
Age					
65–74	1.207*	1.010	0.649***	0.810	0.563***
	(1.002–1.453)	(0.823–1.240)	(0.531–0.793)	(0.633–1.036)	(0.428–0.740)
75–84	1.347**	2.150***	0.630**	0.903	0.336***
	(1.101–1.649)	(1.716–2.693)	(0.506–0.784)	(0.694–1.175)	(0.242–0.466)
85+	2.252***	4.117***	0.449***	0.510***	0.396***
	(1.631–3.110)	(2.851–5.946)	(0.330–0.612)	(0.358–0.729)	(0.246–0.637)
Belong to social website					
Yes	1.167	0.952	1.230	0.715*	1.137
	(0.920–1.481)	(0.733–1.236)	(0.953–1.589)	(0.520–0.985)	(0.816–1.583)
Sexual orientation					
Heterosexual	0.988	0.778	1.134	0.920	1.063
	(0.728–1.342)	(0.553–1.094)	(0.825–1.558)	(0.630–1.345)	(0.668–1.93)
Highest qualification					
Degree	0.619***	0.574***	0.726**	0.425***	0.913
	(0.514–0.746)	(0.466–0.706)	(0.595–0.887)	(0.332–0.545)	(0.673–1.241)
A-level etc.	0.643***	1.163	0.838	0.640*	1.270
	(0.490–0.843)	(0.857–1.578)	(0.625–1.122)	(0.450–0.912)	(0.862–1.872)
GCSE etc.	0.635***	0.708**	0.986	0.709*	1.201
	(0.513–0.786)	(0.559–0.898)	(0.784–1.241)	(0.538–0.936)	(0.873–1.652)
Place of residence					
Urban	1.165	1.134	1.169	1.151	0.750*
	(0.984–1.380)	(0.940–1.370)	(0.978–1.398)	(0.926–1.430)	(0.579–0.972)

(Continued)

Table 10.3 (Continued)

Covariates	Long-standing illness or disability (% yes) Model 1	Health limits moderate activities (% yes) Model 2	Satisfaction with health (% dissatisfied) Model 3	Health status (% poor health) Model 4	General happiness (% not happy) Model 5
Long-standing illness					
Yes		6.798*** (5.724–8.073)	2.294*** (1.929–2.728)	4.738*** (3.766–5.961)	1.652*** (1.216–2.246)
Health limits activities					
Yes			3.178*** (2.673–3.780)	4.513*** (3.657–5.568)	1.180 (0.885–1.575)
Satisfaction with health					
Dissatisfied				3.982*** (3.285–4.827)	2.747*** (2.089–3.612)
Health status					
Poor					1.845*** (1.395–2.440)
Model Chi-square	84.55***	780.22***	480.87***	1265.23***	268.02***
df	9	10	11	12	13
−2 log likelihood	3955	3393	3689	2705	2045

Note: Statistically significant at *$p < 0.05$, **$p < 0.01$, ***$p < 0.001$. Odds ratio (OR) for reference category (ref.) is 1.000.

urban sample and the results show a statistically significant relationship with health outcome ($p < 0.001$). Therefore, geographical location may be important in terms of availability of resources and social networks. Long-standing illness or disability increases dissatisfaction level of health as many as 2.294 times ($p < 0.000$, 95% CI: 1.929–2.728). This implies that disability issue is very important for women living alone and further research can be done to explore this area. Those whose health limits moderate activities are found to have positively associated with health dissatisfaction (OR = 3.178***, 95% CI: 2.673–3.780). In this paper, we have developed an empirical model (Model 4) where health outcome is dichotomy (1 for poor health and 0 for others). Our analysis shows that the higher the age the poorer is the health status. Belonging to social network lowers the risk of reporting poor health and it is found to be statistically significant. Higher education is linked with lower reporting of poor health and this is found to be statistically significant in Table 10.3. Variables – suffering from long-standing illness or disability, if health limits modern activity and if dissatisfied with health – all are strongly associated with reporting of poor health. Modelling heath status is common in health and social science literature (Khan and Raeside, 2014; Khan and Flynn, 2015).

Finally, Model 5 was constructed to measure general happiness and to capture well-being of individual. The outcome measure used asked the respondents to indicate 1 for not happy and 0 for otherwise. Therefore, fitting a logistic regression seems to be appropriate like others. It has been found that age is strongly association with general happiness or well-being. The results show that the higher the age the lower the propensity of reporting not being happy in the sample. This may be mainly due to the existence of health issues. Those women residing alone in urban areas are less likely not happy (in other words more likely to be happy) than their counterparts living in rural areas. Long-standing illness increases the likelihood of reporting that they were not happy with a 1.652 times higher probability of reporting not being happy. Similarly, dissatisfaction with health and poor health status of individuals are positively associated with not being happy. This indicates that poorer health outcome has increasing effect on not being happy.

Discussion and conclusion

Having a contemporary research agenda which includes the specific need of a diverse group of women within the ageing population is becoming more significant if we are to grapple with the unique challenges of demography. The increasing emphasis on intergenerational relationships; meeting individual needs and developing policies on public health needs to take account of the specific characteristics of cohorts of women whose living circumstances are changing within a more fluid society. Little research has been done on the situation of women living alone and how changing relationship status impacts on their future needs and well-being, particularly in relation to how key public services, such as those providing care and support, may need to respond and develop. As we will see in the next chapter, ageing women who have experienced long-term singlehood and who have not had children are a group of particular risk (Hafford-Letchfield et al., 2016).

This paper aims to generate further discussion by attempting to identify some of the issues that may face ageing women living alone for whatever reason based on nationally representative data available from the *Understanding Society*. There may be limitations in the data available given the complexity of what we conceptualise, understand and try to define as a woman living alone in later life given the different choices, experiences and relationships happening at different stages in the life course (third age, fourth age, etc.). For example, the inclusion and exclusion criteria for defining women living alone are extremely complex and inclusion criteria are mainly around self-selection given the range of measures involved. Researchers will need to develop a range of very complex variables in order to understand the trends of women who are living alone more clearly. This was one of the limitations of our paper in that it was not always possible to isolate the characteristics of single women living alone. They may, for example, include women who have been in unsuccessful or disrupted long term relationships in earlier life, as well as those who may have had unsuccessful pregnancies or infant /child death leading to their single status or in living alone. However, further debate about the relevance of these factors makes it possible to regard them as a separate group within ageing and gender studies and to explore the impact of these different experiences on successful ageing. Limitations, for example, for capturing data that relate to people with diverse sexual and gender identities are already well documented and subject to pressure for urgent reform (Betts, 2009).

The analysis demonstrated that biological age plays an important role across life cycle and is a major determinant of health and well-being status of individuals. Education may be another important variable for women living alone in terms of how they may be able to adjust and cope with the challenges of later life. There were some findings associated with measuring perceptions of health and happiness in this group of women which will need to be interrogated further. The availability of social networks in view of absent familial relationships and thinking about the impact of sexual orientation on the types of 'families' and support networks that older lesbian, gay, bisexual and transgendered people may value, all merit further investigation.

The variables measured in the survey may help understand just some of the possible trends for women living alone in later life and the potential different 'positions' occupied by this group. By looking at variables associated with health and well-being, such as education, long-standing illness, satisfaction with health and health status, we have started to identify some determinants when looking at status within ageing studies. This was by no means conclusive but illustrates the challenges of studying women who meet these criteria. Within the increasing trend of women living alone over time and space, there is a need to adapt and develop more accurate measures and research designs in order to investigate the specific nature of ageing for those who are living alone and the diversity of women within this category. Further research can be done to capture a wider picture which can include qualitative studies to try and evaluate the real strengths and challenges that women are facing or may face in the future alongside a data driven approach.

Key recommendations for applying research to professional practice

- When coming into contact with older people living alone, show awareness and sensitivities to the complexities for the reason why they may be living alone and make space for their biographies to emerge.
- Help older people living alone to access the internet or social media, which may help to increase their social networks and networking capabilities.
- Ensure diversity in your approach to offering support to women living alone in relation to their backgrounds, life stories and future needs.

References

Al-Kandari, Y.Y., Crews, D.E. (2014). Social support and health among elderly Kuwaitis. *Journal of Biosocial Science* 46 (4), 518–530.

Ballantyne, A., Trenwith, L., Zubrinich, S., Corlis, M. (2010). 'I feel less lonely': What older people say about participating in a social networking website. *Quality in Ageing and Older Adults* 11 (3), 25–35.

Banks, L., Haynes, P., Hill, M. (2009). Living in single person households and the risk of isolation in later life. *International Journal of Ageing and Later Life* 4 (1), 55–86.

Betts, P. (2009). *Developing survey questions on sexual identity: Cognitive in-depth interviews.* London: Office for National Statistics.

Bildtgard, T., Oberg, P. (2017). *Intimacy and ageing: New relationships in later life.* Bristol: The Policy Press.

Burch, T.K., Matthews, B.J. (1987). Household formation in developed societies. *Population and Development Review* 13 (3), 495–511.

Byrne, A. (2008). Women unbound: Single women in Ireland. In: Yans-McLoughlin, V. and Bell, R. (eds.), *Women alone.* New Brunswick, NJ: Rutgers University Press, 29–73.

Carr, D. (2004). The desire to date and remarry among older widows and widowers. *Journal of Marriage and Family* 66 (4), 1051–1068.

Demey, D., Berrington, A., Evandrou, M., Falkingham, J. (2011). The changing demography of mid-life, from the 1980s to the 2000s. *Population Trends* 145 (1), 16–34.

Demey, D., Berrington, A., Evandrou, M., Falkingham, J. (2013). Pathways into living alone in mid-life: Diversity and policy implications. *Advances in Life Course Research* 18 (3), 161–174.

DEMOS. (2014). *"A vision for care fit for the twenty-first century": The commission on residential care*. London: Demos.

Dorfman, R., Walters, K., Burke, P., Hardin, L., Karanik, T., Raphael, J., Silverstein, E. (1995). Old, sad and alone: The myth of the aging homosexual. *Journal of Gerontological Social Work* 24 (1/2), 29–44.

Dykstra, P.A. (2009). Childless old age. In: Uhlenberg P. (ed.), *International handbook of population aging*. Dordrecht: Springer, 671–690.

Eurostat. (2002). La Vie des Femmes et des Hommes en Europe, un Portrait Statistique [The Lives of Women and Men: A Statistical Portrait]. Brussels: European Commission.

Gabrielson, M.L., Holsston, E.C. (2014). Broadening definitions of family for older lesbians: Modifying the Lubben social network scale. In: Giunta, N. and Rowan, N.L. (eds.), *Lesbian, gay, bisexual and transgender ageing: The role of gerontological social work*. London: Routledge.

Gaymu, J., Springer, S. (2010). Living conditions and life satisfaction of older Europeans living alone: A gender and cross-country analysis. *Ageing and Society* 30 (7), 1153–1176.

Girling, L.M., Morgan, L.A. (2014). Older women discuss planning for future care needs: An explanatory framework. *Journal of Aging and Health* 26 (5), 724–749.

Hafford-Letchfield, T. (2011). Grey matter really matters: A study of the learning opportunities and learning experiences of older people using social care services. *International Journal of Education and Ageing* 2 (1), 8–23.

Hafford-Letchfield, T. (2013). Social work, social class and later life. In: Formosa, M. and Higgs, P. (eds.), *Social class in later life: Power, identity and lifestyle*. Bristol: Policy Press.

Hafford-Letchfield, T., Lavender, P. (2015). Quality improvement through the paradigm of learning. *Quality in Ageing and Older Adults* 16 (4), 1–13.

Hafford-Letchfield, T. (2016) *Learning in later life: Challenges for social work and social care*. Surrey: Ashgate.

Hafford-Letchfield, T., Willis, P., Smith, A. (2016). In the margins or the mainstream? Future directions and innovations in providing inclusive accommodation and support for older LGBTI adults. *Quality in Ageing and Older Adults, Special Edition* 17 (1), 1–5.

Hank, K., Wagner, M. (2013). Parenthood, marital status, and well-being in later life: Evidence from SHARE. *Social Indicators Research* 114 (2), 639–653.

Heaphy, B., Yip, A. (2003). Uneven possibilities: Understanding non-heterosexual ageing and the implication of social change. *Sociological Research Online* 8 (4), 1–19.

Hosmer, D.W., Lemeshow, S. (2000). *Applied logistic regression* (2nd ed.), New York: Wiley.

Hughes, M. (2009). Lesbian and gay people's concerns about ageing and accessing services. *Australian Social Work* 62 (2), 86–201.

Inglehart, R. (2002). Gender, aging, and subjective well-being, *International Journal of Comparative Sociology* 43 (3–5), 391–408.

Kalogirou, S., Murphy, M. (2006) Marital status of people aged 75 and over in nine EU countries in the period 2000–2030. *European Journal of Ageing* 3 (1), 74–81.

Kharicha, K., Iliffe, S., Harari, D., Swift, C., Gillmann, G., Stuck, A.E. (2007). Health risk appraisal in older people 1: Are older people living alone an 'at-risk' group? *British Journal of General Practice* 57 (537), 271–276

Khan, H.T.A., Raeside, R. (1997). Factors affecting the most recent fertility rates in urban-rural Bangladesh. *Social Science and Medicine* 44 (3), 279–289.

Khan, H.T.A. (2014). Factors associated with intergenerational social support across the world, *Aging International* 39 (4), 289–326.

Khan, H.T.A., Raeside, R. (2014). Between country variations in self-rated-health and associations with the quality of life of older people: Evidence from the Global Ageing Survey. *Applied Research in Quality of Life* 9 (4), 923–949.

Khan, H.T.A., Flynn, M. (2015). Self-reported health status of older adults in Malaysia and Singapore: Evidence from the 2007 Global Ageing Survey. *Applied Research in Quality of Life* 11 (3), 687–705.

Khan, H.T.A., Hussein, S., Rahman, S.M. (2015). *Changing family structures, living arrangements and care support for the elderly in Gulf Cooperation Council (GCC) countries: Some policy implications.* Paper presented at the Doha International Family Institute (DIFI) Annual Conference on "The Arab Family in an Age of Transition: Challenges and Resilience" held at Doha, Qatar, 3–4 May, 2015.

Khan, H.T.A., Leeson, G.L. (2006). The demography of ageing in Bangladesh: A scenario analysis of consequence, *Hallym International Journal of Ageing* 8(1), 1–21.

Khan, H.T.A., Rahman, T. (2016). Women's participations in economic and NGO activities in Bangladesh: An empirical study on the Bangladesh Demographic and Health Survey (BDHS). *International Journal of Sociology and Social Policy* 36 (7/8), 1–25.

Kirkwood, T. (2014). Biological determinants and malleability of ageing. In: Kirkwood, T.B.L. and Cooper, C.L. (eds.), *Wellbeing in later life*. West Sussex: Wiley Blackwell.

Kohli, M. (1999). Private and public transfers between generations: Linking the family and the state. *European Societies* 1 (1), 81–104.

Lahad, K., Hazan, H. (2014). The terror of the single old maid: On the insolubility of a cultural category. *Women's Studies International Forum* 47 (Part A), 127–136.

Laing and Buisson. (2014). *Care of elderly people market survey* 2013/14. London: Laing and Buisson.

Laslett, P. (1994). The third age, the fourth age and the future. *Ageing and Society* 14 (3), 436–447.

Lee, Y., Xiao, Z. (1998). Children's support for elderly parents in urban and rural China: Results from a national survey. *Journal of Cross-Cultural Gerontology* 13, 39–62.

Lee, R. (2003). The demographic transition: Three centuries of fundamental change. *Journal of Economic Perspectives* 17 (4), 167–190.

Légaré, J., Martel, L. (2003). Living arrangements of older persons in the early nineties: An international comparison. *Genus* 59 (1), 85–103.

Macvarish, J. (2006). What is 'the Problem' of singleness? *Sociological Research Online* 11 (3). www.socresonline.org.uk/11/3/Source

Maynard, M., Afshar, H., Franks, M., Wray, S. (2008). *Women in Later Life: Exploring Race and Ethnicity*. Berkshire: McGraw-Hill.

McFall, S. (2013). *Understanding society: The UK household longitudinal study, Waves 1–3, user manual*. Colchester: University of Essex. Institute for Social and Economic Research.

McNair, S. (2009). *Demography and lifelong learning: Inquiry into the future for lifelong learning thematic paper 1.* Leicester: National Institute for Adult Continuing Education.

OECD. (2005). *Society at a glance.* Paris: OECD.

ONS. (2014a). National life tables, United Kingdom, 2011–2013. *Statistical Bulletin,* London: Office for National Statistics.

ONS. (2014b). Estimates of the very old (including Centenarians) for England and Wales, United Kingdom, 2002 to 2013. *Statistical Bulletin,* London: Office for National Statistics.

ONS. (2016) Population ageing and the lives of older people, including ageing indicators such as estimates of the very old (90+ by age and sex), median age and sex ratios at older ages at national and local levels. *Statistical Bulletin,* London, Office for National Statistics.

Pampel, F.C. (1992) Trends in living alone among the elderly in Europe. In: Rogers, A. (ed.), *Elderly migration and population redistribution.* London: Belhaven, 97–117.

Pinquart, M., Sörensen, S. (2000). Influences of socio-economic status, social networks and competence on subjective well being in later life: A meta-analysis. *Psychology and Ageing* 15 (2), 187–224.

Pinquart, M., Sörensen, S. (2001). Gender differences in self-concept and psychologicalwell being in old age: A meta-analysis. *Journal of Gerontology: Psychological Sciences* 56B (4), 195–213.

Porter, E.J., Oyesanya, T.O., Johnson, K.A. (2011). "Hoping to See the Future I Prefer" an element of life-world for older women living alone. *Advances in Nursing Science* 36 (1), 26–41.

Powell, J., Khan, H.T.A. (2013). Ageing and globalisation: A global analysis. *Journal of Globalisation Studies* 4(1), 137–146.

Rahman, M.O., Menken, J., Kuhn, R. (2004). The impact of family members on the self-reported health of older men and women in a rural area of Bangladesh. *Ageing and Society* 24 (6), 903–920.

Rahman, M., Khan, T.A., Hafford-Letchfield, T. (2016). Correlates of socioeconomic status and the health of older people in the UK: A review. *Crisis, Illness and Loss* 24 (4), 195–216.

Reher, D., Requena, M. (2017). Elderly women living alone in Spain: The importance of having children. *European Journal of Ageing* 14 (3), 311–322.

Scharf, T., Phillipson, C., Smith, A.E. (2004). Poverty and social exclusion growing older in deprived urban neighbourhoods. In: Walker, A. and Hagan Hennessy, C. (eds.), *Growing older quality of life in old age.* Maidenhead: Open University Press, 81–106.

Silverstein, M., Conroy, S.J., Gans, D. (2012). Beyond solidarity, reciprocity and altruism: Moral capital as a unifying concept in intergenerational support for older people. *Ageing and Society* 32 (7), 1246–1262.

Sourbati, M. (2004). *Internet access and online services for older people in sheltered housing.* York: Joseph Rowntree Trust.

Thanakwang, K., Soonthorndhada, K. (2011). Mechanisms by which social support networks influence healthy ageing among Thai community-dwelling elderly. *Journal of Ageing and Health* 23 (8), 1352–1378.

Timonen, V., Doyle, M. (2014). Life-long singlehood: Intersections of the past and the present. *Ageing and Society* 34 (10), 1749–1770.

Trais, J. (2016). *The lives of older lesbians.* Basingstoke: Palgrave.

UK Dataservice. (2015). *Understanding society: Waves 1–4, 2009–2013.* Colchester: Essex University of Essex. Institute for Social and Economic Research and Nat-Cen Social Research.

UN. (2015). *World population prospects: Key findings and advance tables.* Working paper No: ESA/P/WP. 241. New York: Department of Economic and Social Affairs, Population Division. United Nations.

Victor, C., Scambler, S., Bond, J., Bowling, A. (2000). Being alone in later life: Loneliness, social isolation and living alone. *Reviews in Clinical Gerontology* 10, 407–417.

Weeks, J., Heaphy, B., Donovan, C. (2001). *Same Sex Intimacies: Families of Choice and other Life Experiments.* London: Routledge.

Wolf, D.A. (1995). Changes in the living arrangements of older women: An international study. *The Gerontologist* 35 (6) 724–731.

World Health Organization. (2006). *Defining sexual health: Report of a technical consultation on sexual health.* Geneva: World Health Organization.

11 Stories of intimacy and sexuality in later life

Solo women speak

Nicky Lambert, Trish Hafford-Letchfield,
Hafiz T.A. Khan, Dominique Brady,
Ellouise Long and Lisa Clarke

Introduction

This chapter presents selected findings from a study on the impact of the rise in non-traditional family relationships on 'successful' ageing. The focus of which is on Solo women – women who are 'not-partnered', without children and who are aged over 50 years and over. Little is known about the life trajectories of Solo women as they move into later life (Darab and Hartman, 2013) and there is a paucity of research seeking to understand their support networks, social connectedness and personal relationships. This chapter draws on selected findings from a study which explores some of the dynamics and issues impacting Solo women in later life using a range of methods including a literature review, demographic analysis, an online survey and interview data. Here we draw principally on the findings from qualitative data from the online survey (see Letchfield et al, 2017) and in-depth interviews with Solo women in England aged 50 years and over. Considered together, these findings captured a rich picture of Solo women's own subjective perspectives about the links between their relationship status and well-being in later life - and in this chapter we focus particularly on the findings relating to sexuality and intimacy.

Intimacy in later life

Intimate relationships can shape our sense of self and are linked to positive physical, emotional and psychological well-being (Bildtgard and Oberg, 2017). However, most knowledge about intimate relationships centres around our early and middle years and the importance of understanding later-life intimacy can be overlooked. However, as social mores have changed over the last 20 years, more academic literature has begun to emerge exploring older people's attitudes towards sexuality in later life (see Simpson et al., 2016; Gewirtz-Meydan et al., 2018) and this research is beginning to inform our conceptualisation of sexuality and intimacy in care settings and continues to change expectations in regard to best practice (Hafford-Letchfield, 2008; Simpson et al., 2016). This evolving landscape poses opportunities and challenges for governments, policy makers and service providers in the context of responding to a recognition of the needs of diverse demography. Our findings are discussed in the context of this wider picture and we conclude with recommendations for practitioners in relation to how we encourage and facilitate the voices of Solo women in order to design and provide tailored support to meet their unique needs.

Defining Solo

A diverse range of terms have been used to describe the relationship status of women aging without children and unpartnered in the research so far (Rice, 1989; Wengar, Scott and Patterson, 2000; Wenger, 2001; Cwikela, Gramotnevc and Lee, 2006; Allen and Wiles, 2013; Beth Johnson Foundation, 2016). However, much of the terminology suggests a deficit position (i.e. 'childlessness') and has a tendency to perpetuate heteronormative discourse about familial relationships. Whilst the term 'Solo' for women can be challenging, it is a genuine attempt to describe women's life experiences in a non-pejorative way in the face of language which fails to reflect the shifting political and social circumstances impacting on demography and the impact of gender and sexual inequalities. Such language often lacks sensitivity to a variety of parenting circumstances, i.e. participants with stepchildren, foster children and even estranged children, whilst other studies view people with stepchildren or adopted children as parents (cited in Allen and Wiles, 2013).

Indeed, further analysis of childlessness has resulted in the categorisation of types of childlessness, such as 'voluntary' (childfree) and 'involuntary' (childless), synonymous with 'childless by choice' and 'childless by circumstances' respectively (Connidis and McMullin, 2012). These concepts have also been associated these with measures of psychological well-being and regret (Jeffries and Konnert, 2002; Reher and Requena, 2017). Moreover, in assessing psychological well-being, distinctions are made between never having a child and having lost a child through traumatic circumstances, although both may involve a sense of loss.

Another example of conceptual ambiguity, the term 'singleness' is likewise problematic, in that this may indicate having never married or been in a cohabiting relationship as well as including those who have been no longer married, such as the divorced or widowed. It also includes those in the lesbian, gay, bisexual and transgender (LGBT) community who, for legislative reasons, were prohibited from forming traditionally recognised partnerships earlier in their life (Hafford-Letchfield, 2014). In addressing this, researchers acknowledge that 'partnership status is dynamic' (Simpson, 2016; Hoestler, 2009) and reflects diversity and changes in the patterns of relationships over the life course. Whilst there is a lack of consensus in defining these terms to study Solo women in later life, our approach to the study has been one of self-definition which invited women to identify and describe their own status in relation to the phenomenon (Hafford-Letchfield et al., 2017).

Demographic context

The study of gender issues within ageing populations is of major interest globally given that women represent just under half of the population (Powell and Khan, 2013). Understanding the different life trajectories and diversity characteristics of the ageing female population is important in part because of the implications for wider society and culture. Women's changing circumstances, attitudes and behaviours affect their experience of ageing at both an individual and societal level, which necessitates governments, policy makers and service providers to rethink their care provision. UK life expectancy for women is increasing year on year (ONS, 2013, 2015) and in parallel the 'traditional' life-stage trajectory is changing (Erikson, 1959).

Shifts in how we have previously conceptualised life stages and lifestyle choices are starting to have a marked impact on the shape, size and types of households in the UK. As indicated earlier, women living alone in later life may be a lifestyle choice as well as the consequences of other influencing factors such loss of a partner (Victor et al., 2007), finding the right relationship at the right time, and the impact of fertility control and fertility problems (Al-Kandari and Crews, 2014). More diversity in relationship status has also been influenced by a preference and the social and financial possibility for women to co-habit, live alone, delay marriage, divorce and separate if they wish to (Victor, 2010), not to mention the fluidity and dynamics which characterise post-modern 'liquid' relationships (Bauman, 2003; Klinenberg, 2012). Women are therefore more likely to find themselves moving into later life without a long-term partner or children.

Further, women's economic empowerment, educational and employment opportunities (Cleland 2002; Lee, 2003; Ogg and Renaut, 2007; Raeside and Khan, 2007), the ongoing achievements of equality legislation and women's rights and the mainstream acceptance of individualism, are further factors influencing the various circumstances which older women may experience during their life courses (Raeside and Khan, 2007; Hafford-Letchfield, 2013).

A significant achievement of feminism, for example, has been to challenge notions of compulsory heterosexuality (Rich, 1980) and particularly the experiences of lesbian, bisexual and transgendered women in relation to their 'families of choice' which are only just beginning to be systematically researched (McCarthy and Edwards, 2011; Traies, 2016). According to Byrne (2008), feministic ideologies positively support constructions of womanhood as married and mother, a context in which singlehood and the opposition between woman identity and single identity are now problematic (p. 29). In the absence of positive and powerful counter narratives, singlehood is disparaged and stigmatised constraining the identity possibilities for all women. Against this background, academic research on 'singleness' is surprisingly sparse and relatively underdeveloped, with few empirical investigations most of which are coming from a feminist discursive analysis (Lahad and Hazan, 2014).

Study design and methodology

This was an exploratory study and our study design incorporated an online mixed methods survey questionnaire comprising of twenty items based outlines findings from a literature review. Thirteen items captured demographic variables on the individual respondents including age, ethnicity, sexual and gender identity, highest level of education, employment status, annual income and whether the respondent identified as being Disabled, a carer and/or whether they were living alone. Two of the questionnaire items deployed Likert scales to measure respondents' agreement or disagreement towards a range of issues that emerged from the literature, for example, lifestyle, choice, friendships, social media and subjective well-being (see Table 11.1).

The remaining five questions aimed at gathering qualitative data reflecting subjective commentary on topics such as the respondents' Solo status, their significant relationships, health and social care needs and to also consult them on subjective priorities for further enquiry. The second stage of the study was based on an invitation to all survey participants to participate in in-depth individual interviews using a broad topic guide with open questions based on themes from the findings from the survey and using a narrative approach. Interviews were conducted in person, by telephone or Skype and lasted between 45 and 90 minutes. They were digitally recorded and transcribed.

Sample

Our target population was women aged 50 years and over (a generally accepted marker of fertility decline) who were living in the UK. The preamble was aimed at women who at the time of completing the survey were neither in a long-term relationship nor living with a partner and who did not have children for whatever reasons. We anticipated a challenge in reaching this target group as they are not easily identifiable, there is no obvious place that they naturally congregate and some Solo women may find their identity stigmatised and resist classification by these characteristics. The inclusion criteria were potentially subjective given the fluid nature of personal relationships and histories of individuals' fertility and childbirth, but our overall principle was one that encouraged self-selection against our stated target population.

Table 11.1 Survey questions

	Statements	Strongly agree	Agree	Neither agree or disagree	Disagree	Strongly disagree
A	I am completely happy with my solo status and do not anticipate anything different in respect of quality of life to those who are not solo	28.1	26.6	18.8	25.0	1.6
B	I am very concerned about the implications of growing older as a solo woman	10.9	34.4	20.3	25.0	9.4
C	I made a conscious decision to live a solo lifestyle	25.0	15.6	21.9	29.7	7.8
D	I experience significant mental health issues as a result of being a solo woman	0	9.2	16.9	24.6	49.2
E	My solo lifestyle has caused me to be disadvantaged because of attitudes in current society towards those who do not follow traditional family relationships	7.8	26.6	28.1	18.8	18.8
F	I am extremely content and happy with my current lifestyle	32.3	29.2	26.2	9.2	3.1
G	I am satisfied with my economic situation	26.2	36.9	13.8	16.9	6.2
H	My health is better because of my independence from others	12.3	20.0	49.2	18.5	0
I	I am more likely to be expected to care for others because I do not have any children or dependents myself	10.8	21.5	33.8	20.0	13.8
J	People tend not to take account of my needs or recognise my needs as a solo woman	15.4	30.8	35.4	12.3	6.2
K	If I had the choice I would not be living as a solo woman in later life	14.3	34.9	20.6	12.7	17.5
L	I enjoy a good healthy lifestyle as a result of being solo	12.5	28.1	53.1	3.1	3.1

M	I would recommend living a solo lifestyle	14.3	27.0	50.8	4.8	3.2
N	I wish my life had turned out differently	7.8	28.1	29.7	20.3	14.1
O	I would like to be connected more to people and enjoy better quality relationships	10.9	35.9	20.3	14.1	18.8
P	I would like to enjoy more intimate relationships	19.0	34.9	22.2	12.7	11.1
Q	More should be done to support solo women in later life	18.8	29.7	45.3	3.1	3.1
R	I am very satisfied with my intimate relationships	7.9	15.9	44.4	19.0	12.7
S	I enjoy a rich network of support from my relationships with friends	39.1	35.9	21.9	3.1	0
T	I would like to be in a relationship	15.9	31.7	27.0	12.7	12.7
U	I have a lot of regrets about how my life has turned out	3.2	17.7	29.0	29.0	21.0
V	I would recommend my lifestyle and feel that it is enriched as a result of being solo	15.6	23.4	46.9	10.9	3.1
W	I am closer to my family as a result of being solo	10.9	21.9	37.5	20.3	9.4
X	Social media is extremely important to women in my situation	4.7	17.2	48.4	20.3	9.4
Y	There is insufficient support for women living solo	9.4	25.0	53.1	9.4	3.1
Z	I find it difficult to express my needs as a solo woman	9.5	14.3	31.7	30.2	14.3

Procedure

A wide range of methods were used to reach the target population over a period of a year. First by distributing the online survey link to UK networks in touch with older women. A postal and email address was also given to facilitate those who preferred to receive and return a hard-printed copy. Outreach was undertaken to community based organisations working with older women from minority communities to increase inclusivity. This resulted in seven questionnaires being completed face to face by a member of the research team, three of which involved a language interpreter.

Ethical approval was given by the Health and Education Ethical Committee at Middlesex University (Reference: MHESC1404). Participation in both the survey and interviews were voluntary and the data collected was anonymised at the point of collection. The only exception was that the survey respondents were invited to give a name and contact details if they were interested in engaging in a further in-depth interview. This information was removed into a secure separate document then deleted from the data before analysis.

Data analysis

A total of 76 women from the survey were eligible for inclusion. Nearly all of the respondents took up the opportunity to write in the free text commentary boxes in response to the five loosely-structured open questions. These commentaries provided a source of rich qualitative data and covered participants' subjective views on positive and negative aspects of their status, detail about significant relationships and their health and social care needs. From this sample, 23 participated in an individual interview. The qualitative data from both of these sources was abstracted for analysis.

It is important to acknowledge our theoretical positions and values in examining the qualitative data that gave primacy to the women's own description of their realities and to try and understand the phenomenon of "Solo". Thematic analysis can work to "both reflect reality, and to unpick or unravel the surface of reality" (Braun and Clarke, 2006, 3). The use of open coding allowed us to capture issues directly related to the research topic. Data were initially coded at the individual level of each data item by two separate members of the research team, and then the coded data were combined where certain ideas appeared prevalent or latent. The content across the data items was analysed semantically given that data were generated in response to loosely structured questions, resulting in the identification of several categories and themes (see Hafford-Letchfield et al., 2017 for the full thematic analysis of the survey data). Figure 11.1 provides an example of the complexity of the initial coding frame developed as a result.

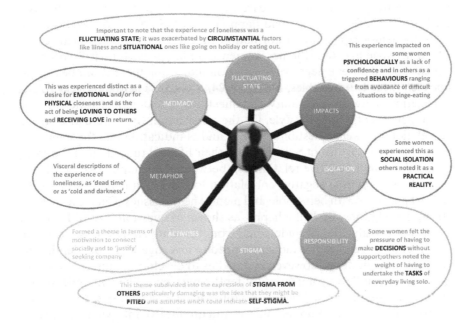

Figure 11.1 Thematic analysis of the survey qualitative data.

Findings

Descriptive data from the survey

Eighty-seven percent of the participants in the sample were between 50 and 65 years. From the 76 respondents, 46 were white British, 6 white Irish, 2 were Asian, 7 African and 8 were from other unnamed ethnic groups. The sample also included 58 heterosexual women and 8 who identified as lesbian, 3 bi-sexual, 1 gender-queer. Four stated that they were undecided and 3 chose not to say. Further, 12 women considered themselves to be either Disabled or 'not sure' if they were Disabled, 52 out of 76 women had graduate qualifications and two had a PhD. Twenty-three women disclosed that they were earning more than £35k per year (above the UK average salary) and 17 with an income of less than £20k per year with the remainder in this middle bracket.

Weightings were given to all positive and negative responses to the series of statements contained in Table 11.1 above which were subject to correlational analysis.

There was no correlation found between being happy with your Solo status and ethnicity, r (63) = −.02, p = .898 nor between sexual identity and being happy with a Solo status, r (63) = .169, p = .189. Similarly, there was no correlation between level of education and happiness with Solo status, r (63) = −.20, p = .117 or income and happiness r (63) = −.01, p = .939.

Furthermore, there was no significant correlation between living alone, r (63) = −.01, p = .912, being a carer, r (63) = .03, p = .819 or being disabled, r (63) = .033, p = .798, and happiness with Solo status. Interestingly, the only demographic type information that was close to significance was found between age and whether women were happy with their Solo status, which showed a weak negative correlation indicating there could be a trend between these two variables, r (62) = −.24, p = .052. There were very strong correlations between question V and questions F, L and all of which discuss the happiness of a Solo lifestyle. On the other hand, there were also strong correlations between question P with K and N indicating that for some they wished that they were not Solo and that their life had turned out differently, also linking to a negative relationship between their happiness with being Solo. Another strong negative correlation found which is interesting is between happiness with being Solo and mental health issues. Choice also had a strong correlation with being happy, as shown in questions C and F. Whilst it was not possible to conclude much from this data source possible due to small sample size, these do indicate a need to investigate in more depth. The value of these findings, however, enabled us to develop our interview schedule within the follow up narrative in-depth interviews. The remainder of this chapter discusses selected themes on intimacy and sexuality from the qualitative data from the combined survey and qualitative interview sources.

Envisioning intimacy

Women's description of their Solo status in terms of their independence versus how they felt being 'alone' was an issue discussed unreservedly by all participants. It reflected a tension that arose constantly in their acknowledgements of the freedoms they also experienced and mostly recognised as a positive one:

> I can leave my hovel messy for days on end and I can do the things I want to do when I want to without having to negotiate or freedom of choice, not having to compromise my own values, not being criticised.

This was posited alongside numerous references to an idealised state which many believed would come as a result of being in a relationship:

> When I have not been in a relationship, it can be feelings of wanting to share quality time with someone. Have someone to do activities with.

This access to another person was also associated with a desire to have someone to provide support:

> There is no one to talk or share with at the end of a working day, particularly if it has been stressful. No-one to give a rational, balanced view.

Others referred to the practical issues of not having someone to help tackle any problems, give advice and the burden of having to make decisions on their own. For some women in the study, closeness had more to do with their pets and they wanted to highlight that the relationship between owner and pet can be extremely significant and 'fill a great void of loving and being loved'.

They spoke about not having a 'ready-made' person to go to local events or on holiday with which would increase spontaneity or reduce the amount of effort they needed to make to socialise. Living Solo also had a cost implication in terms of being responsible for all the routine costs of living and the benefits of sharing costs and having to pay extra on holidays in terms of the single supplement which was identified as discriminatory. Their reference to additional costs associated with Solo status also included the financial implications of always having to be active in making arrangements to socialise, for example, buying tickets for an event or spending money going out for a meal as opposed to being able to socialise at no cost in their own home by 'simply hanging out with someone'. Some of the woman also emphasised the lack of physical contact. Again, there was an idealised version of being in a relationship:

> Well of course, the loneliness. It gets worse as you get older. And I miss closeness, warmth, intimacy, sharing, laughter, loving, compromising…

The temporal nature of living Solo was present in the metaphors that women used, for example, in the image of coming home in the 'winter to a cold house' and times of the year such as during Christmas which particularly triggered a keener awareness of one's own Solo status and having to lie low about their arrangements if they were spending it alone, or not being seen too keen to people who may invite them over to ensure they weren't alone. Whilst sexuality was described along a spectrum from vital to unimportant, intimacy and inversely loneliness were remarked on by most participants. Indeed, women who felt a lack of intimacy described it viscerally in emotional and physical terms. One woman talked about the need for touch and connection as a sensation she called 'skin hunger' saying it was accompanied by a longing to avoid what she called 'dead time' and another woman described her lack of intimacy as a 'cold and darkness' that could not be breached. The desires Solo women expressed were associated with the need to feel closeness, the need for intimacy was at times but not always linked to a wish to be in an intimate relationship.

> …it can be corrosive. Sometimes I would like a hug! I have also got set in my ways in the management of my domestic affairs – partly to ensure the house is clean and presentable without having to spend inordinate amounts of time achieving this result. This means that others can be perceived as obtrusive and disruptive. One needs to find a balance between autonomy etc… and the ability to be welcoming and flexible.

As women were ageing, they felt that their Solo status became more visible which made them feel different or 'on the fringes of life looking in'. They were sometimes subject to unsolicited comments from friends, relatives and by strangers about their Solo status and on occasions even questioned as to why they were on their own at this stage in life. This could provoke feelings of anger and resistance:

> Do not belittle us, just because we are on our own and may sometimes appear eccentric, or anxious, or sad. I held down an incredibly stressful and responsible job but I feel I am now perceived as of no account by health professionals – it is disturbing and infuriating, and isolating.

There were some differences in the data between those who did not choose to be Solo and those who found themselves Solo as a result of their particular life course and circumstances. Hostetler (Hostetler and Cohler, 1997; Hostetler, 2004) suggests that self-determination and permanent single-hood are widely perceived as incompatible. They have questioned whether anyone chooses to be permanently single and what "choice" even means in this context? Many of the participants in the Solo study expressed satisfaction and happiness with their lives although, there was an acknowledgement of the fact that women who would have preferred to have children or partnerships may feel less positive. It follows that someone who has exercised their choice to remain single may feel differently about being Solo than someone who would have liked to be part of a couple and for whatever reason is not. DePaulo and Morris (2006) however describe the phenomenon of 'singlism' – that is bias and discrimination against people who are not in partnerships which may exacerbate this issue. Women noted a lack of a positive public discourse about Soloness and how they were seen as failures in terms of the normative relationships and identities that woman are expected to strive for. Indeed, one woman noted the extreme social discomfort she provoked leading to others conceptualising her as either predatory or tragic.

> ...because of 'other people's perceptions/assumptions lack of a positive public discourse about it [there is an assumption that] you are either trying to shag anything that moves, or sat in the attic with your cats'.

Certainly, though many Solo women were very proactive in seeking connections of all kinds, notably many had extremely full social diaries with memberships of multiple organisations and groups ranging from choirs, faith or cultural communities to educational courses. It should be noted though that some women spoke about feeling disadvantaged in religious groups as single women where notions of the traditional family were promoted and there was a lack of participation from some minority groups for whom being Solo was considered a source social shame.

This vulnerability to the judgement of others also extended to women's own sense of internalised stigma. Mary, for example, deliberately avoids situations where might have to account, or people delve or 'expose' her non-partnered status. She seeks solitude as an escape from the 'chatter going on inside her head' about her situation and the noise of comparing herself to others who are in partnerships. Mary experiences lots of dilemmas in contacting people spontaneously, having to take the initiative to arrange things as well as keeping time for herself.

> My life isn't valued, my lifestyle isn't valued – I need to develop more resilience. I have a different family, mum, siblings etc.

As a black older woman with strong connections to the Pentacostal church, Mary finds intimacy difficult, and tends to keep people at arm's length, is careful not to make any demands, and doesn't allow those in her circle broach the topic of her relationship status. She said that she has a good friend with whom she 'let's slip' sometimes and tends to talk about intimacy in a more intellectual way. There was a fine balance in sharing herself with her friend and not being seen as a burden or raising expectations. Mary also found some comfort in her religious community where the response might commonly be 'that God will provide'. She recently had one episode of acute illness which highlighted for her the importance of knowing who to call or becoming aware of who, if anyone would notice her vulnerability and respond. This resulted in all sorts of insecurities which she said has since triggered her interest in taking care of her own health and keeping well. Mary referred to how some of her networks and family ties had been weakened through immigration and has started to put in places an agreement with other people in church network if they don't hear from each other, then further enquiries will be triggered to ensure someone checks up on them and ensures they are given support.

Mary's situation echoes the interplay between the conflicting images of older women in the media and their lived experience which Solo women in our study explored. Media representations of female ageing are unappealing to most women and this negativity appeared to discourage the Solo women we interviewed from independently generating a positive self-image and recognising that they are part of a growing community of interest. Di Napoli, Breland and Allen (2013) have suggested that the concerns about the sexuality of older, single women seem to be a response from some sections of society fearful of disruption to established family structures as well as a communal anxiety around loneliness and the need for intimacy in older populations. However, ageism and misogyny doesn't allow for the many ways in which post-menopausal women can experience sexuality and intimacy and the importance not just for individuals but for a healthy society of understanding and celebrating the range of desire and connection humans are capable of. One woman stated:

> I have had many good sexual/love relationships. My life as a single woman is wonderful in many ways. I feel very lucky to be living in this time and to have had such a wide range of experiences.

Some women echoed the concern that as their fertility diminished their bodies were increasingly disregarded by professionals. Female health does not appear as high on the agenda as it is in other countries specifically post menopause. Menopause issues are ignored but impact hugely on ability to manage emotional stresses. Muhlbauer and Chrisler (2012) suggest that whilst traditional stereotypes and misconceptions still abound, todays older women has reached maturity with a broader range of experiences and social capital than her forebears. Societal attitudes are yet to adjust to these changes and women on the occasions that they are portrayed in the media can fall foul of stigma directed at both their age and gender (Lemish and Muhlbauer, 2012). In summary, ageing Solo women in this study were well aware of the unappealing nature of the range of personal identities that were socially available to them. Indeed, they felt that these were frequently stigmatised and disparaged; as one participant observed:

> Losing the words 'mad old cat lady' from the language would be an improvement.

Copper (1986), makes a powerful case that western societies elevate the social worth of youth at the expense of older adults. She discusses how since childhood we have been exposed to and have absorbed stereotypes of unnatural aging in women which affect the way we read the bodies of other women and illustrates this with examples of fairy tales built on tropes of wicked witches with unnatural powers which are contrasted with loving, but feeble grannies. But whilst witches are rarely encountered in current public discourse today certainly the concept of older powerful, deviant women is still much discussed in the form of the 'cougar' – a descriptor for older, sexually aggressive women. Whilst, Montemurro and Siefken (2014) welcome the recognition of the possibility of sexual desire and confidence in older women however they note the pejorative use of the image of a sexually incontinent predator to describe an intimate relationship between consenting adults. One only has to look to the media for examples of these conflicts.

Concerns about future care

The concept of intimacy was linked to another theme in the qualitative data concerning the unexplored concerns that Solo women were harbouring about their future care needs. Certainly there were a disproportionate number within the sample who were direct carers for their parents or relatives mostly because their siblings or relations assumed that they would be available to do this because of their Solo status. A couple of women found this experience of caring providing an uncomfortable mirror into their own uncertain futures complicated by the inability to discuss these insecurities with the person they were caring for, for fear of causing them anxieties about what would happen when they were no longer around to provide mutual support.

June, an older lesbian was mostly concerned about older people not being well served by health and social care provision generally but that as a lesbian, her personal context would be further disregarded:

> [Will there be a] respect for my sexuality, for my disposition, for my independence? I think there can be a tendency to see older people, not just women, as a homogenous group.

Almack, Seymour and Bellamy (2010) wrote about the importance of 'families of choice' to LGBT communities, the idea that meaningful, supportive and health sustaining relationships form outside the formal ties of blood or marriage. These connections which can be overlooked by formal health and social care structures must be recognised and supported by professionals (Hicks, 2014; Lahad and Hasan, 2014). Indeed, many women in the Solo study described the essential role of friends in terms of love and relationships as well as in meeting their support needs. It was clear that their friendship is not a lesser form of intimacy, secondary to family or sexual partnerships but a key to living well.

> My happiness as a Solo woman is largely due to my positive attitude and reasonable self-esteem, which is reinforced by my good friends. We support each other in this regard.

Maria who had been forced to take early retirement due to disability had a very tenuous financial situation by the age of 60 years and was dependent on disability benefits and a small pension. She said that she has 'a lot going on' but no one with whom to talk it through. Her only living relative is an elderly aunt who lives 80 miles away, but otherwise Maria had no siblings or parents. She has a few close friends but is very aware of not becoming a burden which could threaten her otherwise good relationships. She therefore contains a lot of her feelings so that she is mostly seen as good company and has someone she can turn to when in a 'real crisis'. Maria highlighted a number of issues about using health and social care and how she saw each part of the service not able to relate to each other and within that context felt that there was no particular person she could talk to about her situation. She desperately wanted to plan for her future and put legal arrangements in place for someone to make decisions on her behalf should her mental capacity become an issue, but currently has no-one to nominate as her ap-pointed advocate. This is something that she perceived could be too much of a responsibility and thus burden to her friends. She belongs to a few groups that meet online and has recently tried dating which has not been successful because of the prohibitive costs and her perception of the competition. She is also unable to have a "traditional sexual relationship because of disability so happy to put that aside". Maria enjoys art based activities that she can do Solo and help her to relax. She is interested in considering a phased supported living arrangement as her needs increase. She felt however that there could be more support networks for older Solo woman and overall saw herself as extremely vulnerable and unsafe and this made her feel very depressed at times. Her main concern was being subject to abuse if she had to enter care without anyone looking out for her.

Crockett, Brandl and Dabby (2015) note that the lack of gender analysis in the field of safeguarding is matched by a lack of a lifespan approach to violence against women. These results in an unclear picture in terms of the numbers of women at risk and who are actively harmed (Brownell, 2015). However, the concerns were broad enough in 2013 for a United Nations re-port to state that violence against older women that it was a policy concern in every region regardless of development level. Violence can be physical, emotional, financial etc. but it can also manifest itself as casual disregard and rudeness sadly from professionals, as well as more generally. One woman described an encounter with her GP; it is disparaging and marked by power imbalances along the lines of class, gender, and not least age.

> I have occasionally found that male GPs tend to view elderly women as a bit of a joke or neurotic which doesn't help. I have even been asked "Why don't you find yourself another man" ... I was able to change my GP immediately after this comment.

Whilst the women experiencing this disrespect were able to identify this dis-crimination as unacceptable and they pro-actively avoiding reoccurrences, they did not report complaining or formally challenging unprofessional at-titudes and behaviours.

Discussion

Relationship status has central significance within policy and drives the way in which we frame the design and future provision of quality care and support. For example, those working directly with older people will be con-cerned to describe the older person's social and economic connections and personal and community networks. Education, health or social welfare pol-icies similarly make many assumptions about family forms, for example, in relation to what is expected from its members, living arrangements; work patterns; financial security including inheritance; and subsequent roles taken up in later life. This is particularly relevant to caring and who is considered qualified to make decisions about older women who might become vulnerable in later life (Hicks, 2014). However, the rise in non-traditional family relationships towards 'families of choice' (Weeks, 2003; Trais, 2012) and growing sociological analysis of practices, discourses, display or enactment previously associated with 'the family', have tried to capture and describe contemporary forms of relationality, intimacy and personal life (see Hicks, 2011; Edwards, Ribbens McCarthy and Gillies, 2012). These important observations about gender expectations as part of the fabric of everyday life and the social nature of expectations of Solo women in particular, should facilitate the deconstruction of ageing experiences so as to understand how policy and practices aiming to support successful ageing might need to develop and respond.

Lifespan developmental theory and research have similarly highlighted the important role of individual choice, control, and self-determination. Indeed, some of the most prominent models of the lifespan place control processes at the center of development (Baltes, 1997; Brandtstädter and Rothermund, 2002). In later life, a time purportedly characterised by flexible roles and freedom of expression (Laslett, 1994) we need to understand in more detail how increasing individual responsibility and latitude in determining life course trajectories is seen across a wide variety of transitions and developmental processes, including the transition to later life (Arnett, 1998) and decisions related to relationship status and ageing Solo (see Hostetler and Paterson 2017).

Demey et al. (2014) found that the relationship history of people living alone in mid-life matters for their psychological well-being. Increasing numbers of people in the UK are living alone in mid-life and rising levels of loneliness and isolation are a concern for the health and social care system as the baby boomers of the 40s and 60s begin to swell the system. This generation has witnessed profound changes in family life. Higher separation and divorce rates mean that many will have complex and diverse partnership trajectories and family networks. Increasing research on the connection between partnership status and psychological well-izbeing has found that the well-being of those living without a partner is lower than those living with a partner. No significant differences in well-being were found between those who had or hadn't lived with a partner. Analysis of individuals who experienced a break up and the effect on them short and long-term and suggested that there might be a longer-term negative effect of experiencing more than one partnership break-up particularly taking into account the financial effect on women in particular. Partnership history and psychological well-being are also affected in different ways by relationship breakdowns, with implications for resilience in later life.

Whilst there are a lot of trends in social relationships, generally the research shows that our day-to-day interpersonal relationships heavily influence our actions, preferences and behaviour and an individual's choices and actions ultimately lead to the cumulative effect on our larger social structure. Social distance can be conceptualised as involving how regularly people interact with others and social structures can be revealed by analysing interpersonal ties and our connections to people. Social distance between people can be measured in terms of a wide range of social categories such as educational level, occupation, ethnicity, measures such as leisure and consumption, cultural and spiritual preferences, the sharing of values, attitudes and other lifestyle choices and connections.

Gender is a major determinant of life chances and patterns but there are a number of nuances and complexities in relation to different age cohorts and the intersectionality of ageing issues. Gender is also an important factor in the labour market given the continuing evidence on pay differentials, career patterns. Solo's women working lives may differ significantly from other groups of women who may have a more established pattern of mixing employment with childrearing or have more fragmented careers. Solo women may also work longer and defer retirement if they are non-partnered, perhaps because of the intrinsic attractions of their work, the social contact and status, but also for necessity in order to accumulate sufficient pensionable and retirement income. The tensions of work life balance may also be different as women with childcare may have different pressures where there are economic and social pressures for achieving dual incomes. Strategic planning for ageing is often about priorities for supporting dependency and also public perception of later life is often out of step with reality. Policy around personalisation needs to support more individual decision making and promote skills enabling individuals to maintain their sense of self.

This chapter has sought to introduce readers to the concepts of Solo ageing and gender and has provided some examples from the Solo women study into the impact of relationship status on intimacy and sexuality in later life. We conclude with some ideas that social workers may need to act upon in order to ensure that they recognise this potentially vulnerable group in order to tailor support and promote well-being.

Key recommendations for applying research findings to professional practice

- Use a narrative approach to establish the importance of networks and support when working with women who may be ageing Solo in order to build on their strengths and identify gaps in support.
- Avoid the use of deficit language, for example, 'not married', 'childless' when talking to and about Solo women.
- Consider the impact of multiple and cumulative losses when working with Solo women that may impact on their mental health and seek out any relevant networks that might not be immediately obvious, for example, where they have experienced infertility or loss of a child earlier in life.

- Utilise legislation and policies in relation to advanced care planning to discuss Solo women's future care needs.
- Ensure that any assessment and support recognises and capitalises on Solo women's resilience and help them make links to community based organisations where needed.

References

Al-Kandari, Y.Y., Crews, D.E. (2014) Age, social support and health among older Kuwaitis. *Quality in Ageing and Older Adults*, 15 (3), 171–184.

Allen, R.E.S., Wiles, J.I. (2013) How older people position their late-life childlessness: a qualitative study. *Journal of Marriage and Family*, 75 (1), 206–220.

Almack, K., Seymour, J., Bellamy, G. (2010) Exploring the impact of sexual orientation on experiences and concerns about end of life care and on bereavement for lesbian, gay and bisexual elders. *Sociology*, 44 (5), 908–924.

Arnett, J.J. (1998) Learning to stand alone: the contemporary American transition to adulthood in cultural and historical context. *Human Development*, 41 (5–6), 295–315.

Baltes, P.B. (1997) On the incomplete architecture of human ontogeny: Selection, optimization, and compensation as foundation of developmental theory. *American Psychologist*, 52 (4), 366–380.

Bauman, Z. (2003) *Liquid Love: On the Frailty of Human Bonds*. Cambridge, Polity Press.

Beth Johnson Foundation and Ageing without Children (AWOC). (2016) *Our Voices: The Experiences of People Ageing without Children*. Leicester, Beth Johnson Foundation.

Bildtgard, T., Oberg, P. (2017) *Intimacy and Ageing: New Relationships in Later Life*. Bristol, The Policy Press.

Brandtstädter, J., Rothermund, K. (2002) The life-course dynamics of goal pursuit and goal adjustment: a two-process framework. *Developmental Review*, 22 (1), 117–150.

Braun, V., Clarke, V. (2006) Using thematic analysis in psychology. *Qualitative Research in Psychology*, 3 (2), 77–101.

Brownell, P. (2015) Neglect, abuse and violence against older women: definitions and research frameworks. *South Eastern European\Journal of Public Health*, 27 (5), 410–421.

Byrne, A. (2008) Women unbound: single women in Ireland. In: Bell, R. M. and Yans, V. (eds) *Women on Their Own: Interdisciplinary Perspectives on Being Single*. New Brunswick, NJ, Rutgers University Press.

Cleland, J. (2002) *Education and Future Fertility Trends, with Special Reference to Mid-transitional Countries*. New York, UN Population Bulletin.

Connidis, I.A., McMullin, J.A. (2002) Sociological ambivalence and family ties: a critical perspective: a critical perspective. *Journal of Marriage and Family*, 64 (3), 558–567.

Copper, B. (1986) Voices: on becoming old women. In: Alexander J. (ed) *Women and Aging: An Anthology by Women* (pp. 46–57). Corvallis, OR, Calyx Books.

Crockett, C., Brandl, B., Dabby, F.C. (2015) Survivors in the margins: the invisibility of violence against older women. *Journal of Elder Abuse and Neglect*, 27 (4–5), 291–302.

Cwikela, J., Gramotnevc, H., Lee, C. (2006) Never-married childless women in Australia: health and social circumstances in older age. *Social Science & Medicine* 62 (1), 1991–2001.

Demey, D., Berrington, A., Evandrou, M., Falkingham, J. (2011) The changing demography of mid-life, from the 1980s to the 2000s. *Population Trends*, 145 (1), 1–19.

DePaulo, B.M., Morris, W.L. (2006) The unrecognized stereotyping and discrimination against singles. *Current Directions in Psychological Science*, 15 (5), 251–254.

Di Napoli, E.A., Breland, G.L., Allen, R.S. (2013) Staff knowledge and perceptions of sexuality and dementia of older adults in nursing homes. *Journal of Aging and Health*, 25 (7), 1087–1105.

Edwards, R., Ribbens McCarthy, J., Gillies, V. (2012) The politics of concepts; family and its (putative) replacements. *British Journal of Sociology*, 63 (4), 730–746.

Erikson, E.H. (1959) *Identity and the Life Cycle: Selected Papers. Psychological Issues*. New York, International Universities Press, Inc.

Gewirtz-Meydan, A., Hafford-Letchfield, T., Benyamini, Y., Phelan, A., Jackson, J., Ayalon, L. (2018) Ageism and Sexuality. In: Ayalon, L. and Tesch-Roemer, C. (eds) *Contemporary Perspectives on Ageism Series: International Perspectives on Aging*. New York Springer International. Open Access.

Hafford-Letchfield, T. (2008) What's love got to do with it?: developing supportive practices for the expression of sexuality, sexual identity and the intimacy needs of older people. *Journal of Care Services Management*, 2 (4), 389–405.

Hafford-Letchfield, T. (2013) Social work, social class and later life. In: Formosa, M. and Higgs, P. (eds) *Social Class in Later Life: Power, Identity and Lifestyle*. Bristol, Policy Press.

Hafford-Letchfield, T. (2014) Social work with lesbian, gay, bisexual and transgendered older people. *Community Care Inform Adults*. ISSN 0307-5508.

Hafford-Letchfield, T., Lambert, N., Long, E., Brady, D. (2017) Going Solo: findings from a survey of women aging without a partner and who do not have children. *Journal of Women and Ageing*, 29 (4), 321–333.

Hicks, S. (2011) *Lesbian, Gay and Queer Parenting: Families, Intimacies, Genealogies*. Basingstoke, Palgrave Macmillan.

Hicks, S. (2014) Deconstructing the family. In: Cocker, C. and Hafford-Letchfield, T. (eds) *Rethinking Anti-discriminatory and Anti-oppressive Theories for Social Work Practice*. Basingstoke, Palgrave.

Hostetler, A.J. (2004) Old gay and alone: the ecology of well-being among middle-aged and older single gay men. In: De Vries, B. and Herdt, G. (eds) *Gay and Lesbian Aging: Research and Future Directions* (pp. 143–176). New York, Springer Publishing Co. Inc.

Hostetler, A.J. (2009) Single by choice? Assessing and understanding voluntary singlehood among mature gay men. *Journal of Homosexuality*, 56 (4), 499–531.

Hostetler, A.J., Cohler, B.J. (1997) Partnership, singlehood, and the lesbian and gay life course: a research agenda. *International Journal of Sexuality and Gender Studies*, 2 (3–4), 199–230.

Hostetler, A.J., Paterson, S.E. (2017) *Toward a community psychology of aging: a lifespan perspective*. In: Bond, M. A., Keys, C., and Serrano-Garcia, I. (eds) *Handbook of Community Psychology*. Washington, DC, American Psychological Association.

Jeffries, S., Konnert, C. (2002) Regret and psychological well-being among voluntarily and involuntarily childless women and mothers. *International Journal of Aging and Human Development*, 54 (2), 89–106.

Klinenberg, E. (2012) *Going Solo: The Extraordinary Rise and Surprising Appeal of Living Alone*. New York, Penguin.

Lahad, K., Hazan, H. (2014) The terror of the single old maid: on the insolubility of a cultural category. *Women's 520 Studies International Forum*, 47 (Part A), 127–136.

Laslett, P. (1994) The third age, the fourth age and the future. *Ageing and Society* 14 (3), 436–447.

Lee, R. (2003) The demographic transition: three centuries of fundamental change. *Journal of Economic Perspectives*, 17 (4), 167–190.

Lemish, D., Muhlbauer, V. (2012) "Can't have it all": representations of older women in popular culture. *Women & Therapy*, 35 (3–4), 165–180.

McCarthy, J.R., Edwards, R. (2011) Families of choice. In: McCarthy, J. R. and Edwards, R. (eds), *The SAGE Key Concepts Series: Key Concepts in Family Studies* (pp. 57–59). London, Sage Publications.

Montemurro, B., Siefken, J.M. (2014) Cougars on the prowl? New perceptions of older women's sexuality. *Journal of Aging Studies*, 28 (3), 35–43.

Muhlbauer, V., Chrisler, J.C. (2012) Women, power, and aging: an introduction. *Women & Therapy*, 35 (3–4), 137–144.

Ogg, J., Renaut, S. (2007) The influence of living arrangements, marital patterns and family configuration on employment rates among the 1945–1954 birth cohort: evidence from ten European countries. *European Journal of Ageing*, 4 (3), 155–169.

Office for National Statistics (ONS). (2013) *Cohort Fertility, England and Wales, 2011. Statistical Bulletin*. London, ONS.

Office for National Statistics (ONS). (2015) *Trends in Life Expectancy at Birth and at Age 65 by Socio-economic Position Based on the National Statistics Socio-economic Classification, England and Wales 1982–1986 to 2007–2011*. Statistical Bulletin. London, ONS.

Powell, J., Khan, H.T.A. (2013) Ageing and globalisation: a global analysis. *Journal of Globalisation Studies* 4 (1), 137–146.

Raeside, R., Khan, H. (2007) The ageing Scottish population: trends, consequences and responses. *Canadian Studies in Population*, 35 (2), 291–310.

Reher, D., Requena, M. (2017) Elderly women living alone in Spain: the importance of having children. *European Journal of Ageing*, 14 (3), 311–322.

Rich, A.C. (1980) Compulsory heterosexuality and lesbian existence. *Journal of Women's History*, 15 (3), 11–48.

Rice, S. (1989) Single, older childless women: differences between never-married and widowed women in life satisfaction & social support. *Journal of Gerontological Social Work*, 13 (3–4), 35–47.

Simpson, R. (2016) Singleness and self-identity: the significance of partnership status in the narratives of never-married women. *Journal of Social and Personal Relationships*, 33 (3), 385–400.

Simpson, P., Almack, K., Walthery, P. (2016) 'We treat them all the same': the attitudes, knowledge and practices of staff concerning older lesbian, gay, bisexual and trans residents in care homes. *Ageing and Society*, 1–31. doi:10.1080/01634372. 2011.585392.

Traies, J. (2012) Women like that: older lesbians in the UK. In: Ward, R., Rivers, I., and Sutherland, M. (eds) *Lesbian, Gay, Bisexual and Transgender Ageing: Biographical Approaches for Inclusive Care and Support* (pp. 76–82). London, Jessica Kingsley Publishers.

Traies, J. (2016) *The Lives of Older Lesbians*. Basingstoke, Palgrave.

Victor, C. (2010) *Ageing, Health and Care*. Bristol, Policy Press.

Victor, C., Scambler, S., Bond, J., Bowling, A. (2000) Being alone in later life: loneliness, social isolation and living alone. *Reviews in Clinical Gerontology*, 10 (4), 407–417.

Wenger, C.G. (2001) Ageing without children: rural wales. *Journal of Cross-Cultural Gerontology*, 16 (1), 79–109.

Wengar, C.G., Scott, A., Patterson, N. (2000) How important is parenthood? Childlessness and support in old age in England. *Ageing and Society*, 20 (2), 161–182.

12 Sexuality, gender and intimacy, reflecting on professional practice

Priscilla Dunk-West and
Trish Hafford-Letchfield

Introduction

In this edited collection, we have explored aspects relating to sexuality, intimacy and gender which are under-theorised in social work. For many scholars, sexuality has been neglected, not only in mainstream social work research, but also in social work education. In this chapter, we examine some of the key gaps in knowledge and consider ways in which professional education might respond to such gaps. First, we trace some of the key findings of the research showcased in each chapter and explore the utility of using a life course approach to understand sexuality, intimacy and gender.

In Chapter 1, we outlined the rationale for the presentation of the material contained in this book. One of the key points we made was that the use of the life course lens offers a way to view human experience: from childhood to older age. Given the issues that have been uncovered in this edited collection, such an approach demonstrates that people of all ages encounter issues related to relationships, intimacy, gender identity and subsequent inequalities. We argue that social work has much to offer people throughout the life course. Although social work is often conceptualised in relation to fields of practice, or specialisms, we contend that for too long, issues relating to identity such as sexuality, gender or intimacy have been viewed as the domain of specialised knowledge. Seeing relationships, intimacy and gender—which are at the core of human experience (Dunk, 2007)—as 'outside' the scope of social work does a disservice to the knowledge that social workers have and relegates such knowledge to the 'other'. We argue that social work, as a profession, ought to include knowledge in its curricula, which speaks to these important dimensions to human experience. Second, social work is committed to working to promote equality and to actively challenge oppression in its remit towards social justice. Sexual and gender minorities continue to face inequalities and oppression in a range of ways. For example, the intersections between other aspects of social life and identity such as race and religion have an impact on the ways in which homophobia is expressed and experienced (Magrath, 2017). Many social commentators would note the rise of alternative narratives to the negative portrayal of same sex attraction and identity. The 'it gets better' video is an example of the use of temporal narratives of 'success' of lesbian and gay people, though some researchers argue that such discourses of 'success' replicate classism (Meyer, 2017). What is important is that social research in the area of gender and sexual diversity is that this kind of research demonstrates a commitment to social justice:

> If our profession's commitment to diversity, social justice and multiculturalism are to have more than rhetorical significance, we have to find ways of defining these terms clearly and carrying out our scholarly and educational activities in the context of this philosophical orientation.
>
> (Reisch, 2013, p. 728)

As well as understanding the interaction between other aspects of identity, this edited collection is important in the ways in which research questions relating to gender, sexualities and intimacy are framed.

Social researchers are interested in social phenomena. Similarly, it is important that social work and social care research draws from the complex ways in which social conditions, knowledge about power and inequality and the commitment to social justice come together in the framing of research questions. Not only must research about sexuality and gender be undertaken, it must be informed by social justice principles. Thus, the selection of the research contained in this edited collection has been informed by asking: what areas that are under theorised and whose voices are missing? This edited collection is therefore crucial to the contemporary landscape in which complexity between social conditions and identity are intertwined. The role of the 'mission of social work' is central to this project, not least because:

> In adapting to neo-liberal discourse, revised means of conceptualizing, producing and disseminating knowledge, research and evidence have been introduced with little assessment of their potential effects on the long-standing mission of social work and the character of practice and education.
>
> (Reisch, 2013, p. 721)

Of course separating out gender and sexuality from other aspects of identity decontextualises each from the social conditions within which they are named and categorised. In Chapter 2, we see this by understanding role that the social plays in determining what gender categories have become normalised through the lens of conformity. In this chapter, the focus is on gender non-conformity in children. The role that institutions play in regulating the role of gender is examined in Chapter 3. In this chapter, the issue of homophobic and trans bullying was investigated and found to be a major social issue. Chapter 4 drew from the emerging recognition that intimacy is not confined to sexual or romantic relationships. Friendships are a kind of 'sociable resource' (Tsai, 2006) and have been demonstrated to affect the sexual behaviours of young people (Byron, 2017). The expansion of intimacy to non-sexual relationships is an important shift in social research and Chapter 4 examines the role that intimacy plays in the social relationships defined as friendships. In Chapters 5–8 adulthood is examined in relation to gay men, transgender people and their intimate relationships and sexual identity in the workplace. The concept of relationship satisfaction is also examined: all of these issues relate to the personal, interpersonal and consider the role of space, whether work or the domestic sphere. Chapters 9–11 consider the experiences of older people and outline the role of togetherness, being solo and being intimate in older life. In each chapter of this edited collection, researchers have asked questions pertinent to gender, sexuality, intimacy and relationships: what do they mean to people? What experiences do people have that need to be understood in the broader social context? What role does inequality play in the experiences of people? Importantly, the authors have considered: what factors are important for professionals to know about? Before moving on to consider the educational needs for social workers and other professionals, let's take a look at the utility of the life course approach and the reason for the use of such a framework in this edited collection.

The life course approach can be conceptualised in two ways. First, it is an approach which we have used in this book to demonstrate the ubiquity of issues relating to sexuality and gender at varying points throughout one's lifetime. Although social work services are arranged according to particular sectors, the professional role that might be of assistance in childhood, adolescence, adulthood and later life are important to consider in relation to what skills and knowledge are needed for social workers and other helping professionals to have in relation to working with issues of gender, sexuality, intimacy and relationships. Second, such a framework can be used to imagine an individual's trajectory in life, from birth to death. The experience of being gender non-conforming in childhood, for example, may impact on future experiences and opportunities throughout adolescence, adulthood and later life. This kind of application of a life course perspective seeks to illuminate oppressive forces and structures pertinent to a particular life stage. Longitudinal research is useful in this sense: it points to the need for early intervention and resource allocation early in the life stage. For example, recent research has found that girls who were given increased opportunities to access education and books in early life were more likely to be in paid work during adulthood (Majeed, Forder, Mishra, Kendig, & Byles, 2015). Such seemingly individual experiences must not be separated from the broader social conditions in which life is experienced. The rise of communicative technology has been identified for some time by sociologists as shifting our experiences into new ways of relating (Lash, 2001). We face new challenges brought about by shifts in contemporary relationships, couple and family configurations and expressions of intimacy (Gabb & Fink, 2015). This has implications for the ways in which social workers and other professionals are educated:

> During the past several decades, a 'perfect storm', comprised of economic globalization, a dramatic demographic and cultural transformation, and rapid technological advances, has created unprecedented challenges for the social work profession and social work education.
>
> (Reisch, 2013, p. 716)

Social work education must respond to the needs of its service users: professionals working with people will likely encounter issues relating to gender, sexuality, intimacy and relationships. This requires professionals to exercise skills and knowledge about such issues. More specifically, the life course approach offers a way to frame such issues. This includes:

- The conceptualisation of gender in childhood and understanding of non-conformity and social expectations around gender
- The role of institutions in reproducing gender categories and conformity such as schools and other services which children and their care givers encounter
- The ways in which sexuality is expressed in early adulthood and adolescence
- The meanings of intimacy and friendships for young people
- The role of education as an institution as a potential source through which inequalities are produced
- The rituals, meanings and expressions of relationships in middle adulthood
- The role that institutions such as the workplace and domestic sphere play in middle adulthood in relation to gender, sexual identity and relationships
- The expressions of relationship categories in later life
- The role that institutions play in constructing heteronormative structures, potentially silencing bisexual, lesbian, gay and queer identities

There is much to be done to continue research in the area of gender, sexuality, relationships and intimacy. As social forces continue to shift into the future, the voices of people who have not been included in research must move into the foreground. Social justice ought to inform this kind of research into the future: education for professionals must equip its workers to remain up to date and literate in the ways in which the people with whom they work. This edited collection is therefore an important contribution to the practitioner, student and teacher of professionals. Research contained in this book speaks to the heart of the professionals, harnessing the narratives of those whose voices are often silenced.

References

Byron, P. (2017). Friendship, sexual intimacy and young people's negotiations of sexual health. *Culture, Health & Sexuality, 19*(4), 486–500. doi:10.1080/13691058. 2016.1239133

Dunk, P. (2007). Everyday sexuality and social work: Locating sexuality in professional practice and education. *Social Work and Society 5*(2), 135–142.

Gabb, J., & Fink, J. (2015). Telling moments and everyday experience: Multiple methods research on couple relationships and personal lives. *Sociology, 49*(5), 970–987. doi:10.1177/0038038515578993

Lash, S. (2001). Technological forms of life. *Theory, Culture & Society, 18*(1), 105–120.

Magrath, R. (2017). The intersection of race, religion and homophobia in British football. *International Review for the Sociology of Sport, 52*(4), 411–429.

Majeed, T., Forder, P., Mishra, G., Kendig, H., & Byles, J. (2015). A gendered approach to workforce participation patterns over the life course for an Australian baby boom cohort. *Journal of Vocational Behavior, 87*(Supplement C), 108–122.

Meyer, D. (2017). "One day i'm going to be really successful": The social class politics of videos made for the "it gets better" anti-gay bullying project. *Critical Sociology, 43*(1), 113–127. doi:10.1177/0896920515571761

Reisch, M. (2013). Social work education and the neo-liberal challenge: The US response to increasing global inequality. *Social Work Education, 32*(6), 715–733.

Tsai, M.-C. (2006). Sociable resources and close relationships: Intimate relatives and friends in Taiwan. *Journal of Social and Personal Relationships, 23*(1), 151–169.

Index

access to services 16
affirming approach 19
ageing capital 70
ageing without children 177
ageism 81
ambivalence 77

bisexuality 142; and ageing 145; knowledge
    gaps 146; lifecourse perspectives
    144–145; theoretical perspectives 143
Bourdieu, Pierre 69, 70, 73
bullying: causes 41; definitions 31, 32;
    faith based 29; parental engagement
    42–43; peer support 43; prejudice
    driven 31; prevention 41; social media
    42; transphobic 34; types of 40

care needs 188–90
caring 75, 76, 189
childlessness 177
cisgender patriarchy x
cisgenderism 86, 91
clinician engagement 98
coming out 101, 105
compulsory heterosexuality178
corrective rape ix
covert discrimination 109
cultural constraints 78

disclosure 103
diversity management 101
DSM-5 17, 104

education: good practice 35
embodiment 87
enduring love 121, 129
Erikson 178

families of choice 69, 70, 189
feminism 72, 96, 143, 178–179
fetishisation 86

friendships: boundaries 61; categories/
    typologies 49; characteristics 54;
    friendship families 71; gender
    differences 50; language used 60–61;
    performing/doing/displaying 58, 63;
    rituals and symbols 51–52; soulmates
    50; theoretical perspectives 49

gay: homemaking practices 73; scene 69
gay village 78
gender: and ageing 156, 192;
    discrimination 109; dysphoria 86,
    88; identity 14; kinship 71; non
    conforming 11; queer 11; variant 11

Henrickson, Mark xi
heterosexism 28, 104, 106–109, 112
heterosexuality 3, 5, 69, 72, 74–75, 79,
    81, 93, 101, 104–105, 109
homophobia/homophobic: ageist 81
    bullying 29; EU policy 28;
    harassment 35
HRT12

ILGA 28
intimacy: cisgenderism 86; definition 3;
    in later life 176–77; maintenance of
    56–57; young women 49

labels15
lesbian ix, 3, 19, 27–28, 69–77, 94, 101,
    142–143, 150–151, 157, 160, 163–165,
    170, 177–178, 183, 189, 198, 200;
    lesbian community 92–93; lesbian
    employees 101–103, 106, 108–109,
    110, 114; lesbian parents 31, 33,
    35–37, 52
LGBT history month 36; employment
    101; inequalities at work 109
life stages, lifecourse 178, 191, 200
living alone156, 159

loneliness 107
Looking Both Ways 145

medication 16
minority stress 104

negotiating intimacy 92
non-binary 11
non-monogamy 78
normative intimacy 94–95

online gay scene 80–81
online relationships164

parents of non-conforming
    children 14

quality of relationship scales 122–127
queer ix
queer homemaking 69

race 16, 22, 32, 41, 73, 77, 79, 81–82,
    126, 131, 143, 197
RAINBOW-HAS 29
rejection 14
relationship quality scale 138–139
resilience 14, 71

Section 28 29
sex work 13
sexual identity 3; minorities x;
    orientation 25, 27, 32, 33–34, 38,
101–105, 107–109, 112, 114–115, 126,
    130, 138, 143, 145, 159, 160, 163–164,
    169–170
sexual orientation monitoring 104
sexuality, definition 3
singleness 177
singlism 186
social class 74
social justice x, 144, 151, 197–200
social work: and bisexuality 144;
    family support 20, 44;
    Federation 21; homophobic
    bullying 45–6; International
    interventions 17; practice 3, 4,
    71, 115, 139, 142–143, 146; Solo
    women 176
soulmates 50
Stonewall 32, 37
suicide14

trans: youth 11
transgender intimacy 86
transgender partners 97
transition: at work 106; legal obstacles 12;
    medical 11, 88, 92
transphobia 20, 51, 106, 114–115

understanding society 155, 159–60

Weeks, Jeffrey 68, 157
wellbeing 104, 155
workplace discrimination 102

Milton Keynes UK
Ingram Content Group UK Ltd.
UKHW040101071024
449327UK00019B/706